DR. HER
PONI
AGE-OLI
CAN M

"In their way, they love as much and as little as women do, even though the traditional evaluation standards of relationships suggest that women are the love connection. If women want to love men, they will need first to know men's reality and their impact on that reality. This book challenges women to go beyond their explanations and responses to men and to look through men's eyes and inner reality. The best of men's love potential has not yet begun to be tapped."

In this ground-breaking book, Dr. Herb Goldberg reveals how men and women can really understand and enjoy each other without all the misunderstandings and the anger. WHAT MEN REALLY WANT should be required reading for every woman who loves a man . . . and every man who wants a closer, more intimate relationship with a woman.

HERB GOLDBERG is one of America's most widely read psychologists. In addition to his best-selling *The Hazards of Being Male,* Dr. Goldberg is the author of three books on men's psychological health, *The New Male, The Inner Male,* and *The New Male-Female Relationship.* All three are available in Signet editions. He is a clinical psychologist practicing in Los Angeles, where he also makes his home.

WHAT MEN REALLY WANT

by

Herb Goldberg

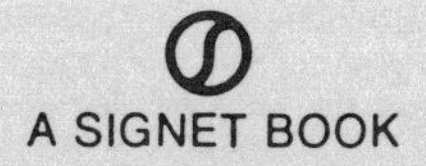

A SIGNET BOOK

SIGNET
Published by New American Library, a division of
Penguin Putnam Inc., 375 Hudson Street,
New York, New York 10014, U.S.A.
Penguin Books Ltd, 27 Wrights Lane,
London W8 5TZ, England
Penguin Books Australia Ltd, Ringwood,
Victoria, Australia
Penguin Books Canada Ltd, 10 Alcorn Avenue,
Toronto, Ontario, Canada M4V 3B2
Penguin Books (N.Z.) Ltd, 182–190 Wairau Road,
Auckland 10, New Zealand

Penguin Books Ltd, Registered Offices:
Harmondsworth, Middlesex, England

First published by Signet, an imprint of New American Library,
a division of Penguin Putnam Inc.

First Printing, June 1991
20 19 18 17 16 15 14 13 12 11 10

Printed in the United States of America

Books by Herb Goldberg

Creative Aggression
(with George R. Bach)

The Hazards of Being Male

Money Madness
(with Robert T. Lewis)

The New Male

The New Male-Female Relationship

The Inner Male

What Men Really Want

Author's Note

In all of the case histories cited, the author has used fictitious names and described traits not identifiable as those of any particular person or persons.

Contents

WHAT MEN REALLY WANT

Introduction

As a writer of relationship books, I have often heard it said that men are fearful of commitment and are insensitive partners. While I agree that it is common for men to have serious deficiencies in the area of personal relating, these very same relationship limitations make them yearn for and open to a committed relationship when they are related to realistically.

Without a close relationship with a woman, most heterosexual men's personal lives are painfully empty and present an unknowing danger to their well-being. Intense hunger and deprivation of personal contact build in them, and they become prone to extreme and self-destructive behaviors and decisions in their pursuit of satisfaction and relief from their isolation and need for close contact.

Most women are unaware of the enormous potential power they have in their relationships because of men's need. What this means is that successfully relating to men is potentially very simple once that relationship is rooted in an accurate reading of the man and his relationship experience and reality.

Women go to great lengths to make themselves physically appealing to men. Although being "beautiful" may initially attract a man's attention, what holds and binds him is the sense that his partner really likes and wants him and that her interest and desire are based on knowing his true inner self.

Men sense intuitively, even though they may not be consciously aware, when a woman's feelings are genuine and not just designed to satisfy her need for a committed relationship. In the latter instance, he "knows" it is just a matter of time before she will begin to confront him with his deficiencies, try to change him, and blame him for all the problems in the relationship.

Establishing a close relationship with a man is enormously frustrating, if not impossible, for the woman who carries negative interpretations and stereotypes of men in relationships. The woman who cannot see men objectively, acknowledge the impact of her negative predispositions, and take responsibility for the effect of her reactions on the understanding and solving of mutual problems, will be creating her own self-fulfilling prophecy. That is, her relationships will produce pain and turmoil partially because her inability to relate to men realistically is triggering men's defensive and insensitive behaviors rather than bringing out their loving potential.

Women can establish relationships with men in two ways. The most common one has been through the use of feminine ploys and sexual allure. Using feminine power to excite and tie a man to her, however, has a steep price. These relationships are initially romantic and exciting, but become distant and abusive. Men's behavior in these relationships becomes defensive as they get caught up in a cycle in which they sense they are not accepted and loved for the person they know themselves to be; they become cold and hostile in response.

The second way to establish and develop a relationship is by gaining an accurate understanding of a man's strengths and limitations—what he can and cannot give in a particular situation, and the combined effects of his and her relating. When that occurs, and love and caring still remain, the relationship has achieved a strong foundation for growth and depth.

If I have succeeded in my intent, this book will provide a psychological map for the development of a realistic and authentic relationship. While writing this book, I found myself working hard to avoid justifying or romanticizing men as persons in need of understanding, who have a great untapped potential for love. Nor do I believe that the burden of making a relationship work should be placed on the woman. Rather, I have described what I hope is a useful and accurate portrayal of the male, so that women can relate to men realistically and successfully.

I invite a sharing of reactions and input from both women and men that may provide me with even greater definition of the man-woman relationship condition. I wish you a realistically rooted, happy relationship experience.

HERB GOLDBERG, PH.D.

1

Nothing Personal: The Inner Relationship Experience of Men

> The quantity of love that an ordinary person can stand without serious damage is about 10 minutes in 50 years.
>
> —*George Bernard Shaw**

Chris works as a consultant to the boat-building industry. When a major boat project encounters an unusual problem during construction or if a finished boat turns out to have a complex mechanical flaw and a determination has to be made as to how best to remedy it, Chris and his team are called in.

Chris has an almost psychic ability to get to the heart of the problem with malfunctioning objects by "empathizing" with them. He can "feel" what's wrong—in an automobile, a computer, or a household appliance. It's as if he can diagnose the distress of objects with uncanny detailed accuracy by making himself an extension of them.

Because of this mechanical talent, Chris earns a great deal of money. In a trade magazine for the boat construction industry, he described to

*Bernard Shaw, *The Pursuit of Power, 1898-1918*, Volume II, by Michael Holroyd. Random House, 1988, 1989.

an interviewer how he problem-solves a particularly difficult case. "I can sit on a dock, after walking through the boat, and 'feel' my way into its heart, until the solution comes, often without using diagnostic equipment. I can just tell I'm right even though my notions sometimes sound ridiculous at first to others. I'm rarely wrong."

This ability to identify with the inner workings of an object in distress is matched only by his equally great inability to empathize with or understand the people close to him: his two children by two different wives; the ex-wives themselves who often become infuriated by his insensitivity; and the women with whom he has been involved in the years since his second marriage broke up, who eventually become angered by his mechanical, detached demeanor and his logical approach to the relationship. For example, when a problem arises in the relationship, Chris reacts in a seemingly unfeeling, analytic way to cut through responses he considers irrational. Although he may be superficially correct in his dissection of the words, he misses the essence of what the woman is trying to convey about her feelings and what he is doing to frustrate her and make her feel isolated.

The same women who end up hating him are initially irresistibly drawn to him and are eager to have sex with him when they first begin dating, even though he takes great pains not to pressure them. The endings of these affairs are usually as sudden and extreme in the frustration and breakdown of communication as the beginnings are characterized by excitement, joy, passion, and seeming openness. Of course, none of this makes sense to Chris's logical mind. How can women who seem to love him so much initially, turn on him in anger and frustration when he is sure he hasn't changed. He is convinced women are crazy.

Each time it happens, Chris is left bewildered and confused by the sudden and extreme changes. "I don't understand it and I don't think I'll ever get used to it. I'm honest about where I am from the beginning; I don't push the sex and I don't change, but their feelings sure do. The more I try to get them to know me as I am so that we can have a friendship, no matter what happens to the romantic part, the more I seem to fail. The anger they feel is so strong, I don't think they are hearing anything I'm saying. I give up on trying to be friends with a woman, and I don't believe they're sincere about really wanting to get to know me, have me be myself, and get really close."

As a man, Chris has performed at the highest standards of masculinity, achieving and winning consistently, but his personal life is a shambles. After many failed attempts at love, he has become increasingly fearful of getting involved in a new relationship. Nothing in his personal life works out or survives, even though he believes that he is doing everything right. His career and financial affairs thrive, so he devotes most of his time to them, although he is beginning to feel less fulfilled. Chris feels lost and stuck in his best intentioned efforts at love and relating.

Chris is one of the many men who find themselves defeated in their attempts to relate successfully and intimately to women. Making what they believe are their best efforts, they nevertheless end up being resented or rejected by the women with whom they thought they did everything right. Indeed, today's best-seller lists include many books written for women, concerning men who "can't love" and "hate women," and are either selfish sexists; misguided, pathetic wimps; workaholics and selfish lovers; or abusive addicts. *Most men cannot understand or relate to the accusations. They don't see themselves and their experience the way that women do. When they try to communicate what they do feel, they often make things even worse.*

As a psychotherapist who has worked with many couples, I see how women get fixed negative stereotypes of the man, and a woman's sense of pain, frustration, hurt, and anger prevents her from seeing or hearing what the man is responding to or experiencing, why he has behaved as he does, and the loving things he does. Like the early feminists who were so enraged at men that they became resistant to any alternative perspective, many women with whom I have worked have felt so wounded by the man in their life that the only acceptable solution was for the man to change. They feel they have given until they can't give any longer to a man who has taken but not given in return. Since he couldn't change without his partner also changing, the relationship's end became inevitable.

At the beginning of these relationships, romantic feelings keep things going. He believes that everything will work out and that he is really understood and loved. But when things start to unravel, and his efforts to make himself known and accepted fail, he gives up trying to make himself heard, convinced that talking will not help. He becomes one of the "silent," "closed off" males.

The many books that describe men in a negative light obviously strike a responsive chord in many women or they wouldn't be so successful. The missing ingredient in these books, however, is an accurate and objective depiction of the forces that compel and motivate men; what opens men up and shuts them down, so that women who want to love the reality of the man, the way he experiences himself, can succeed.

The way men love, and what they need in a relationship, are different, and often the opposite of what women need. Indeed, men's needs in relationships, for better or for worse, because of their conditioning as men, have been to suppress and deny vulnerability and personal needs, to avoid losing control or getting too close. Historically, men who didn't have intimate needs were considered the most manly because all of their energy could be focused on doing and achieving. They were taught that that would be enough to make them lovable.

Patrick, a financial consultant, age fifty-five, retired from his investment firm. He was sitting alone in his antique-filled hillside home recuperating from an almost fatal heart attack. He found himself reluctant to ask anyone he knew—women or men—to run some errands for him or to come over and stay with him during his recuperation.

He struggled with loneliness, anxiety, and indecision. "I'm uncomfortable asking anyone to do things for me," he acknowledged. "Maybe it's too much of a commitment to make myself vulnerable that way—to let someone know I need them. The women might get the wrong idea and think it's an invitation to get too close, and I'm not ready for that. If I ask my men friends, they might say no, and then I'll get angry or hurt and maybe I'll never want to talk with them again. I don't want to risk that." So he sat alone, hoping someone would call and the problem would solve itself.

In the hospital's intensive care unit a few days after the attack, Patrick had his "moment of truth" and realized how alone he was and how his best efforts at developing a support system with those he cared about had failed. To be in control and to keep from depending on anyone, he'd put a distance between himself and many of those he really cared about. There was nothing personal in his life and it was frightening to him to acknowledge how he had deluded himself into believing he had been a lovable person.

Patrick was a victim of a socialization that made him a successful, attractive man in the outside world from an impersonal distance, and an isolated, disconnected one in his personal life. Like many men, he had learned to "stand tall and alone," to do for others, but to keep an emotional distance, which he didn't realize he was doing.

Ironically, the "ideal man" in our society is a poor candidate for "being close, loving, and intimate" in the way most women define these traits. He has a long way to grow in awareness and personal change to alter the self-defeating patterns in his personal life. Thus the same man who is initially admired risks being resented and rejected for the personal deficiencies that develop in tandem with his external, impersonal competence.

In their way, Chris and Patrick did all the "right things" a man is taught he's supposed to do to make himself lovable. When they tried to convey their feelings to others, they failed. Then, their tendencies to hide their feelings increased, and the frustrations in communicating with their lovers eroded the relationships.

Over the years I have had the opportunity to work professionally with and get to know the inner selves of many of these men—intelligent, successful, and sensitive in their own right, who "couldn't help" doing well in the competitive world, at the same time they couldn't help entering into painful, convoluted, and destructive interactions with the important women in their lives. Their logical, objective communication talents that worked well for them in their professional lives were not only ineffective but alienating. Their best efforts at loving became lost in the eyes of their partners. Only their deficiencies were apparent.

The personal histories and experiences of these men, and many others as well, follow a similar course. Initially they tried to do everything they were taught was supposed to be responsible and loving. Eventually they reached an impasse. Things didn't work out or frequent arguments and conflict occurred. Initially feeling responsible and wanting to have a successful relationship, each tried to change himself and behave in ways he thought might improve the situation, but eventually failed. Love turned to frustration, which turned to escalating pain and anger until these men found themselves helpless and unable to stop the spiraling, frustrating pattern and make their loving feelings and intentions known.

Do they want things to go badly? Did they plan to make their partners unhappy or to behave in ways that would alienate and anger them? As one man expressed it, "Even my sincerest efforts at being 'nice' seemed to get misunderstood, and I'd find myself being told that I was hostile, or acting in patronizing, dishonest, or manipulative ways. When I would joke or be playful to lighten things up, often I was told I was making fun of the woman or being sarcastic and hurtful. When I'd try to talk things out rationally or explain myself, it only made things worse because I was told I was intellectualizing and being cold and distant. Nothing short of agreeing with her way of thinking, and asking forgiveness seemed enough. Even then I was in a double bind, because apologizing would make me seem weak and intimidated. Going silent and being cold and withdrawn seemed the only solution. She'd be upset at my lack of openness but at least our differences had a bottom line. She could only guess at what I was feeling or thinking."

Was this man the victimizer, the victim, or part of an unfortunate, uncontrollable process in which he was clearly confused and failing in his best efforts to relate in loving ways? Few men want to be isolated, withdrawn, and unloving. To the contrary, the desire to have a close working relationship with a special partner is a matter of urgency for most men because of the absence of personal, caring relationships in a life geared toward achieving, competing, producing, and succeeding.

At the same time, there is no question in my mind regarding men's contribution to the destruction of personal relationships and the pain women experience in them, nor am I implying men are the victims. Intuitively, men must know how difficult and unsatisfying it is to get close to one of their sex, because few men relate to each other personally. Few have close male friends. As a psychotherapist, experienced in the response patterns of men, I have seen even the brightest men in serious crisis with their entire personal lives at stake, unable or resistant to opening up and talking about their feelings.

Marty, a San Diego attorney, comes to mind. A driven businessman in his mid-forties, he had narrowly avoided death as a result of lung cancer, had serious problems relating to the almost grown children of his broken marriage, and had deep feelings of distrust and anger toward women because of an expensive, rancorous divorce battle and a subsequent affair with a woman who abandoned him during a time when his business was failing.

Marty was considering marrying a woman he called his "soul mate," someone he said made it possible for him to fully trust and be vulnerable with for the first time in his life. To his dismay, he found himself experiencing premature ejaculation.

He sought therapy, but found it very difficult to describe or examine his emotions, the details of his inner experience, or his various feelings toward the woman he said he loved deeply. He knew his "sex problem" was emotional because he had undergone physical testing that proved his "sexual equipment," as he called it, was functioning well. Despite his anxiety and concern over the meaning and effect of his problem, and his desire to make the relationship work, he could sustain only a few hours of psychotherapy before closing up and deciding he would work it out by himself. Consequently, the marriage to the love of his life lasted less than a year. His partner finally gave up in total frustration over his inability to talk about the problem and his self-centered, defensive, and controlling attitude—patterns Marty could not recognize or change by himself.

Even with high stakes, and in the throes of despair and anxiety, the resistance to opening up is so automatic and strong for most men that the process of trying to get close to a woman is a struggle. Men don't believe that they can be vulnerable and be treated with loving compassion.

In their personal lives, most men are deficient in the ability to tune in to what those around them are experiencing and feeling. Their energy is focused on outside goals and concerns. At the same time, they tend to deny that any significant problems even exist, until the situation worsens.

This is the critical difference between men and women in their approach to problems. Women seem able to acknowledge their need for help. Men's interpretation of events often leads them to view problems as coming from mistakes, rather than as resulting from an ongoing, repetitive pattern of interaction, in part because of *how* they relate.

Their socialization has "externalized" them to the extent that they are unaware even of being out of touch with their inner selves. So, in the process of becoming successful or achieving, their personal lives become chaotic and dysfunctional. They seek the logical answers and mechanical solutions that work in the outside world, but they fail to find them.

In this way, they operate in relationships "blind." They are rarely intentionally insensitive, unfeeling, or hurtful. In the area of personal relationships, pop psychology and pop spirituality would have us believe that we can be anything we want to be, but for most men that is absolutely not true. They cannot will themselves to be different. In most instances, they can't even frame the problem accurately. Further, they are oblivious to the depth and endurance of the rage they inspire or the ways they are being related to by those who need them, yet fear or dislike them. They continue to believe that they are loved and lovable.

They rationalize their emotional isolation and obsession with building fortresses of security and self-protection as being necessary for survival. They don't question their own poor logic in the face of constantly pursuing the control and security that are never enough to make them actually feel safe. Their approach to personal problems is to provide answers and truth—and to convince others. They are unaware that no one is really listening, even though they may pretend to be.

A well-known psychologist with a national radio talk-show concerning mental health and personal relationships believed he was beloved by family and friends, even though he openly engaged in extramarital affairs. He rationalized that monogamy was prudery and such sexual repression was unhealthy. He told himself that his children and family friends, as well as his wife, benefited from his "courage" and "risk taking," and his commitment to living free, and still respected and loved him.

His reasonable arguments justifying sexual "freedom" were cogent and compelling. What he couldn't see, despite his professional expertise, was the extreme conflict, anxiety, rage, and humiliation that family members felt but were too intimidated to confront him with directly. They hated him for what he did, but they never told him.

While he preached openness and authenticity in relationships over the airwaves, he couldn't see how *the way he related* led to alienation from his family. When his wife divorced him, and ill health forced him to retire, he found out how others really felt about him. Still, he was unable to see how he had brought on the apathy and lack of caring and attention. Instead, he complained bitterly that others were self-centered and had only used him, which was partially true. One truth he could not see was how his defensiveness had blinded him to the way he had participated in creating the lack of caring he was confronting. He had traded being right for being loved, pursuing his abstract visions of life while alienating himself from others.

No question about it. Men need to grow and change. As their personal lives unravel, they are at a loss to understand why, or how to correct it. The personal lives of many men are like a ticking time bomb that could explode at any time—and they can't see it coming.

The problems created by the conditioning of

men are extreme, but are made far worse because of the rage induced in women who harbor intense needs, expectations, and romantic fantasies about closeness that *cannot* be fulfilled, not because the man doesn't want to but because he can't. The ways he is able to love, *by doing for*, do not generate the love or bonding he believes will occur. He feels embittered when he discovers that his best efforts have failed to generate love.

Milton comes to mind because, as a self-made, successful businessman who worked hard all his life, with a credo of not stopping work until he had a minimum of $1500 a day in orders for a line of promotional goods, he entered his fifties with a damaged relationship with his children, and a wife who had committed suicide. All the years of hustling to give his family what he never had not only came to naught, but had inspired rage in his family, who regarded him as abrasive, arrogant, and totally self-centered.

If men were aware of their impact, would they choose to alienate and enrage those close to them—a process that results in their being a major victim also, the alienated member of the family?

A woman's "blind spot" in her personal interaction with a man is comparable to a man's unawareness of his personal impact on others and their feelings. Most women believe that a man acts as he does because he doesn't really care about the feelings of others.

Finding one's way through the mutual misreadings so that men and women can understand one another and the way their responses are actually experienced by the other, and the ways we distort or overreact to what we hear, is the crucial challenge and an indispensable part of a starting point.

We can all see what is being done to us. Few of us, however, are able to see our own impact and participation in creating the response we receive. Men feel as misunderstood, victimized, and exploited as women do, once they can examine the situation objectively. They feel equally as oppressed as women do and are equally as anxious to achieve a successful love relationship.

Miriam, married for twelve years, was angry because her husband would fall asleep at family dinners with her parents, and because he was "cruel" during his discussions with their sons. She did not listen when he told her that the weekly dinner ritual with her parents depressed him and was bad for his health, because he felt he had to eat the rich food and had to listen to her father's critical comments about how he conducted his business. During conversations with the children, she would encourage them to "stand up to" their father and always sided with them.

Miriam's anger about her husband's abrasive manner and "insensitivity" prevented her from regarding his reactions as anything but self-centered justifications. The perception of her husband as intentionally hurtful insured that no constructive change could occur. In couples therapy, when she was able to listen to his interpretations of the events without negative judgments, his response at these family affairs changed dramatically. His positive emotions began to emerge, and his negative tendencies receded.

The way a woman relates to a man can radically affect the degree of his insensitivity, his ability to care, and the way he responds to her assertions.

Although the conditioning of men creates massive personal "blind spots," a woman's inability to understand the impact of her reactions on the man widens the gap and exacerbates their problems. As he feels misunderstood and unfairly blamed and provoked—and then badgered—his worst chauvinistic behaviors emerge.

Many women don't understand a man's intentions. A man who uses his logic and reason to convince a woman of the validity of his perception is hapless and misguided. He is *not*, however, deliberately being cold, distant or antagonistic—all the things she is likely to think he is being—any more than the woman who asks for a hug or who becomes tearful during an argument is trying to manipulate, control, or smother the man—which is how he may misinterpret her response.

The gap must be closed between what men intend by their responses and the way that women perceive and interpret them if men and women are to communicate as caring friends rather than defensive counterparts, convinced the *other person* is responsible for the relationship's problems.

It is my hope that women who are not committed to a negative vision of men will someday write books for men—teaching them to interpret and understand women's responses, with an accurate analysis of how women's responses may be a part of the reciprocal problem of communication so that both can change.

Bringing the reality of men to women and women's negative responses to a neutral starting point so that accurate, objective listening can replace the defensively filtered distortions that now occur, is the purpose of this book. I hope that someday we can look back on this "nightmare" period of mutual accusation and increasing defensiveness, when the relationship between the sexes was being engulfed by distortions, projections, accusations, mutual exploitation, denial of one's own overreactions, and the poisonous "gender undertow," or defensively polarized needs of men and women, and see it as having been a problem caused and solved by both sides.

Men's withdrawal; women's need to be close; men's need to control; women's loss of boundaries; men's "cold" logic; women's "hot" emotionality—are all parts of the defensively polarized cycle that has made modern male/female communication as dangerous as it is alluring. When a man says something in a playful manner that is construed as hostile, or when a woman says something meant lovingly and he construes it as pressuring, the undertow is poisoned. Nothing short of draining it of its defensiveness will bring men and women together in a love based on reality. Both are victims. Both are victimizers. Both have a reality that is not being recognized. Both have an effect on the other that is denied. Both are participating in a precarious, escalating cycle of distorted communications.

We have tried but failed to improve male/female relationships by pointing out each other's sexism and flaws—or believing that a perfect, "magical partner" who is out there somewhere will make it all better. We have been stuck at a point where each sex feels exploited, manipulated, and oppressed.

When euphoric romance—which is the way

most relationships begin—is transformed into alienation and mutual revulsion, until the very sight of one's former partner generates hostility, we are all victims. When the seemingly most compatible of couples feel themselves strangled by, damaged, and unable to control a negative spiral, *the common enemy* of unconscious provocation, misperception, and polarization must be acknowledged and transformed.

Women have made it clear that they do not want their experience and reality defined and interpreted by the men who control the professional, economic world. Men are awakening to their own personal reality and needs in their rejecting the notion that they are the sole source of the personal problems. In the process, they are working to define their own experience and reality in it. Yet their efforts will fail if all they are left with is a sense of righteous rage over being misunderstood, exploited, and abusively treated. Both sexes need to learn about the inner experience of the other.

As women began the process of reclaiming their rightful place in the business world, the relationship between men and women in the "outside world" became better balanced. Similarly, as men reclaim their needs in the personal world and their recognition of their inner self, intimate relationships will improve.

To love and be loved means to know and be known as we really are. Relationships that will thrive in the future are those rooted in realistic mutual perceptions. Denial and fantasy are the hallmarks of romantic fusion that have brought us to the inevitable end points of rage and alienation.

Improving male/female relationships is not merely a matter of resolving issues, but of altering reciprocal rhythms and cycles of communication, understanding each other's limits and intentions, and responding to the other person's experience and intention, as well as his or her impact. Confronting each other about "relationship crimes" and sexism may be a respite from the harder job of seeing how we are each equal contributors to the relationship cycles.

In this book, I hope to connect with the inner voice in each woman that knows men don't bond with women to abuse and control them, and that men and women are trapped in defensive webs of which both have been victims.

In a society where love is freely chosen, questions of whom we choose and how the relationships evolve can teach us most about who we are. We are who we attract and are attracted to. There are no accidents in the intense fusion of romantic bonding. Only the most defensive of us—man or woman—will continue to believe we are victims of unfortunate choices of partners.

Can men love? In their way, they love as much and as little as women do, even though the traditional evaluation standards of relationships suggest that women are the love connection. If women want to love men, they must first know men's reality and their impact on that reality.

This book challenges women to go beyond their explanations and responses to men and to look at men through men's eyes and inner reality. The best of men's love potential has not yet begun to be tapped. The worst of their chauvinistic tendencies are *nothing personal.*

2

The Making of a Man

SHE: Men enrage me! Their self-centered insensitivity and their need to control everything.

HE: But who made them that way? Mothers bring up little boys and have all the power and influence in the early years. Most dads are hardly around. If women want men to change, why don't they blame mothers—go after the hand that rocks the cradle and shapes the little boy?

SHE: Women are controlled by their husbands and by a male-dominated society. The values of that male-dominated atmosphere are so overpoweringly negative they prevent women from having any influence.

HE: That is, unless it works for them. Women complain about the male-dominated society but then want the aggressive, ambitious winners for husbands and lovers. They encourage the worst in men and then complain about it. They shy away from the "softer" man.

SHE: Men's cruelty doesn't make sense. They seem to enjoy being destructive for the sake of it. They destroy everything that gets in the way of their goals.

HE: When it works for them, women applaud it or close their eyes to it. Women reject men who are weak or show fear. That's what's screwing up the little boys; all those double messages: You want them to be "all boy," but then you hate them for being "all man."

SHE: If men got more involved with parenting they'd understand what it's all about.

HE: Most men would get involved in parenting if women could carry the financial load, and if women took their careers seriously enough so that a man wouldn't have to worry that, all of a sudden, she won't want to work anymore and it's poverty time because he didn't pursue his career hard enough because he trusted she'd stay with hers.

SHE: Always the negative response. What is it that makes you guys so pessimistic and cynical?

The Importance of Understanding Who and What He Is

For a man, the worst part of being in what is supposed to be a loving relationship is feeling blamed, accused, or resented for being who he is and has been taught to be; and for doing what he was taught are the proper things to do. For a man who believes he is acting out of loving and caring motives to be told he is selfish, unfeeling, and uncaring, is a major step toward hopelessness and alienation, and the eventual destruction of the relationship.

Intimacy is not possible between people who are unaware of the deeper motivations, realities, and limitations that are the determining core of the person. Understanding him is a critical cornerstone, not just of seeing him as he is but also for a woman to see how she impacts on and affects the man she wants to love.

The Specific Components of His Masculine Undertow

A cluster of unconsciously defensive reactions gives a man the feeling and appearance of being "A MAN." *The more extreme they are, the more manly he appears, but the harder he is to relate to personally.* These components also generate the best and worst of being a man; that best comes at the expense of, and creates, the worst.

Because the "best" of being a man is developed at the expense of the development of his inner or personal self, men are most attractive when at the greatest personal distance, specifically when performing rather than relating and being close and intimate. Women who are irresistibly drawn to these men by their attractive masculine facades soon discover that the intimate relationship aspects turn out to be as painful as the impersonal aspects are attractive. The "worst" of him emerges when he is pressured for personal intimacy he doesn't understand. Therefore, toward the end of a deteriorating relationship, cold, distant, angry, controlling, and closed-off "self-centered" behaviors emerge in the extreme. Conversely, in the best of times, such as in the romantic beginnings when there is little or no stress, these negative defensive tendencies do not surface because they are not being triggered. In a balanced relationship, the distressing coldness and detachment of men are rarely, if ever, present. In extremely polarized relationships, they are always present. The way a woman relates to a man greatly affects whether and how often these responses will occur.

Defensive Autonomy and the Blocking of Dependency

"I can't seem to get close to him"; "I feel like he doesn't really need me"; or "He acts like he just wants to be left alone"—these complaints are the result of a man's defensive autonomy, a major product of his masculine socialization. He acts as if he wants to be left alone, even though he may be unable to cope if he is abandoned. His inner sense of being a man is closely linked to the feeling that he doesn't really need anyone in order to survive.

The wife of an actor, famous for his cowboy roles in which he portrayed independent heroes, described him as "fiercely possessive" in their personal life. Whenever he would go on location to shoot a film, he insisted that she accompany him and leave the children with housekeepers.

Dependency and personal needs are blocked and denied in defensive masculine counterreaction. The more powerful and rigid the counter defense, the more intense the dependent needs he is denying. His desperation and depression when his wife or lover leaves him, and the urgency to be with another woman if he can't get her back, tell us how powerful this denied dependency really is.

What Inner Reality Does Defensive Autonomy Create for Him?

"When the chips are down, you're all you've got. You can't really count on anybody else," and "Nobody really cares," describe his deeper feelings about relationships as a result of his defensive autonomy.

With age this feeling intensifies if he has not had therapy. He is likely to become an isolated and cynical workaholic, busy building up his material security and economic fortress against that "threatening, unloving world" out there. Power-hungry and wealth-seeking men are accumulating protection against a world they see as dangerous and uncaring, unaware of how their *process* creates the nightmare they believe is objective reality.

How Is It Likely to Affect You?

Although initially his defensive autonomy makes him seem strong and attractive, as his partner you will have a frustrating sense that he really doesn't need you, that you are being kept at arm's length and that he never really opens up or allows you to get close. In addition, he may give you cynical sermons about life and the world, attempting to help you become less "naive."

How to Relate to the Effects of His Defensive Autonomy

Seeking reassurance that he needs you is pushing him to acknowledge something that he needs to deny to himself. Maintaining your course and movement toward your separate identity may put the relationship in temporary crisis, but will serve to strengthen it in the long run, and force him to confront his deeper, real needs for closeness.

Defensive Aggression and the Denial of Fear and Vulnerability

The most traumatic and inciteful label to hang on a young boy is "sissy" or "coward." He may risk his life to prove he isn't. The humiliation and emotional scars of these labels will affect and motivate him for a lifetime.

In a polarized intimate relationship, seeming to be "always angry" and easily irritated may be predominant characteristics. Because his reaction is unconscious, it is likely that he doesn't see himself that way. Rather, he may think of himself as lovable.

What Inner Reality Does Defensive Aggression Create for Him?

His defensive aggression makes the world seem like a jungle where one must be vigilant and prepared, and not show fear or weakness. Scratch the surface of an aggressive, power-driven man and you find someone who fears he will be destroyed if he backs down and allows himself to be intimidated. With age, and without therapy, the need to be strong and invulnerable will increase. He "respects" power in other men and reacts critically to weakness, fear, and powerlessness in others as well as himself.

How Is It Likely to Affect You?

As the relationship leaves the romantic phase and he feels undue pressure to be close, he may readily become moody and withdrawn. The more anxious and vulnerable he feels, the more withdrawn and more disconnected he may seem in his unconscious attempt to block these feelings. In addition, the more vulnerable he feels, the more impatient and angry he may seem.

How to Relate to the Effects of His Defensive Aggression

Women who equate love and intimacy with compatibility and an absence of anger may react personally to angry outbursts and irritation. His negative behavior is the result of deeper conflicts and the fears and doubts about himself in the competitive marketplace. Therefore, not reacting to his irritated, impatient comments will help him to see the inappropriateness and offensiveness of his negative moods.

Never tell him to try to be nice or accuse him of always being angry; attempts to cheer him up will not be successful. A straightforward observation that he seems distressed might bring out a positive response. A supportive response that indicates you are not taking his anger and irritation personally is both reassuring and helpful.

Defensive Need to Control (Assertion) and Resistance to Being Submissive (Giving up Control)

He states opinions as truths. He has to be right and he may say defensively, "Nobody tells me what to do or pushes me around." He may dominate conversations and activities or become bored, distracted, and withdrawn if he can't. Proven to be wrong or forced into being submissive may incite hostile responses.

His need to control and to impose his will and opinions alienates and distances those close to him. It is a cornerstone of the personal nightmare he creates for himself as he eventually alienates those who have a personal relationship with him.

What Inner Reality Does His Defensive Need to Control Create for Him?

In his inner reality, it is dangerous to be a loser and allow others to take control. Anxiety over being "nobody" or being told what to do by others causes him to avoid situations that he cannot dominate. Further, it makes him excessively competitive.

The defensive need to control makes it hard for him to ask for help or to seek counseling when he needs it, because it puts him in what he feels is a submissive position, which feels worse to him than his problems. Therefore, he will seek quick, superficial solutions to complex relationship problems.

How Is It Likely to Affect You?

While initially it makes him seem attractive and manly as a self-confident, self-assured person, his need to control is ever-present, and the sense of being unimportant is experienced by those around him. Further, the stress of his need to control and the feeling of not being listened to will create feelings of rage in his partner over being discounted by him. This is a dangerous element in his marriage relationship. This crisis in women's lives when they feel that they can no longer stay married and still be their own person is a common one. Women leave, but men didn't see it coming.

The combination of defensive masculine control and defensive feminine accommodation is lethal in traditional relationships. Women begin to hate men and men distrust women when women "suddenly" change from being "loving" to being "hateful" for what men feel is no apparent reason.

How to Relate to the Effects of His Defensive Need to Control

While men may seem to react negatively to women who have clearly defined preferences, beliefs, and desires, they react far worse in relationships in which they are given control. Maintaining clear boundaries is the most loving thing a woman can do for a man. It prevents her from having a buildup of anger over feeling controlled, and keeps him more fully aware in the relationship because of the ongoing challenge that prevents him from taking her for granted.

Defensive Sexuality and the Repression and Discomfort with Touching and Physical Closeness

Defensive sexuality makes men obsess about sex and is a major cause of relating to women as sex objects. A man's obsession with sex is in proportion to his resistance to personal, emotional contact.

The defensive nature of masculine sexuality drives men to make poor relationship decisions. They are drawn into sexual encounters that are inappropriate or self-defeating.

What Inner Reality Does Defensive Sexuality Create for Him?

Sex and sexual activity become one of his driving forces. His inner reality has the power to make him feel euphoric when sex is exciting, or self-hating and depressed when he can't perform or sex is not available. Sex takes on undue importance as a measure of his self-esteem and as a way to make what he regards as close contact. His sense of being a man and being adequate is linked to his sexual capacities.

How Is It Likely to Affect You?

Initially, a man's intense sexual interest may make a woman feel desirable, feminine, and powerful. Because his interest is defensive and dominant, however, it eventually seems to feel oppressive and offensive. Furthermore, a double-bind is created as she may feel offended by the dominance of his sexual preoccupation but fearful of his losing interest in sex, which translates into personal rejection and a fear that he will turn to someone else.

Mutual "good sex" in traditional relationships is difficult because of men's characteristic discomfort with nongoal-directed physical affection in the form of hugging, kissing, and caressing. Many women feel that the only time a man seems interested in being physically close is when he wants sex, and that turns the sexual intimacy into a negative event.

Men's seeming sexual selfishness results from this defensiveness, and is unconscious. The opposite feeling in him is more likely true—he wants to be a good lover.

How to Relate to the Effects of His Defensive Sexuality

A balanced relationship means a lack of underlying tension and the presence of good sex naturally. A sexually insensitive man cannot be confronted without making things worse. Rather, the focus needs to be on the total relationship; as it comes to involve two people who like each other and relate in a nonpolarized way, his sexual sensitivity will improve. Until that is achieved, the lack of total sexual fulfillment can serve as a guide to how the relationship can become healthy and balanced. In the meantime, accusations about his sexual exploitativeness will only drive a deeper wedge.

Defensive Detachment (Coldness) and the Absence of Feelings

Vulnerable emotions are equated with weakness and femininity. The traditional male seems cold and detached because his approach to life, including personal relationship problems, is to apply logic and analysis. This approach may make him a success in the business world, but a failure in his personal life. It escalates the problem by making the woman feel distanced and impersonally treated.

What Inner Reality Does Defensive Detachment Create for Him?

He fears and distrusts emotional displays in others and in himself. He sees them as manipulative, childlike, and irrational. He becomes convinced that all problems of life must be solved with logic and reason. When others resist he may try to force them to see matters his way. These attempts get "tuned out" by others who experience them as arrogant and insensitive. He concludes that he is surrounded by irrational people and rarely learns from the input he gets. The end result is that he gives up and despairs about having to live in a "crazy world."

He *can't* see how his logic is illogical and how his analytic approach makes things worse and causes him to be hated; and how his "prove it with facts" attitude makes others feel insulted and ignored.

How Is It Likely to Affect You?

While initially his cool, problem-solving approach is comforting because it makes him sound reasonable, the defensive denial of his emotions eventually makes him seem mechanical and unfeeling. His partner will feel distanced and impersonally treated.

Of all the defensive aspects of masculinity, none is potentially more painful than a man's disdain and rejection of the emotions of others in a close encounter. Because he controls his own emotions defensively, he tends to react to tears and emotion with distrust and irritation.

How to Relate to the Effects of His Defensive Unemotional Attitude

He believes he is a feeling person, and in his way he is. Confrontations about his being cold and mechanical only make him feel more misunderstood and angry. Therefore, listening to him and seeing his input as a reflection of his efforts to understand may prevent a polarization.

Although he cannot be pressured to empathize, if less stress exists in the relationship, it becomes easier for him to show loving emotion. The more traditional he is, the colder he seems, although the perceptive woman is aware of the love and attachment he actually feels.

Defensive Goal Focus and the Repression of "Being"

Masculine defensiveness makes him a compulsive doer who needs a goal, purpose, or meaning in order to be motivated and to engage with energy. Defensive goal focus limits his capacity to interact personally for just the pleasure or sake of it. His goal focus puts him out of touch with personal process, so that while he pursues "meaningful activity," he loses awareness of the moment-to-moment aspects of relationships.

What Inner Reality Does Defensive Goal Focus Create for Him?

Anything personal to which he can't assign a purpose or goal he may regard as trivial, boring, or "a waste of time." He feels useful and worthy of being alive primarily when he can "do" and be productive. Consequently, when illness, unemployment, age, or personal problems impair or destroy this capacity, he is prone to feelings of self-loathing, doubt, anxiety, and depression. He feels "useless" and not entitled to enjoy himself and his life when he can no longer perform.

Without a purpose he may become "paralyzed" or unable to function. In personal relationships, when "purpose" is lost, such as after marriage, when courtship is over, he may withdraw and become passive because he is without the goal.

How Is It Likely to Affect You?

Initially his need to do and have a goal makes life interesting. He is planning activities and often wants to try new things. Because the drive is defensive, however, it eventually seems like an avoidance of just being together and a constant pressure "to do."

Even vacations may become onerous because he gets bored without goal-directed activity, and his partner feels pressured to participate with him.

Because he is a defensive doer, he regards those who don't do as lazy and unproductive. This is especially difficult for those who are not compulsive doers like him. Even his approach to solving relationship problems is to "do something" right away.

How to Relate to the Effects of His Defensive Goal Focus

Letting him "do" on his own, without complaining that he seems "unable to just be" and is fearful of intimacy is the most effective approach. At best it will make him pay more attention to your needs. If the desire to be together is not strong on his part, letting him go off "to do" on his own is best for maintaining the relationship, and it may bring him around.

Defensive Disconnection and the Repression of His Inner Self

All of the combined forces of his conditioning pull a man completely outside of himself. The more "a real man" he is the more externalized and disconnected he is. The end points of disconnection are the creation of a seemingly mechanical man, because he is totally outside of himself—a complete performer who relates impersonally and transforms personal experiences into impersonal ones.

Women who are intimately involved with a man get the brunt of his impersonal way of relating and erroneously believe themselves to be singled out to be distanced, when in fact he is reacting to his masculine socialization.

In fact, unconsciously he sees himself as an object by defining himself by what he does and how well he does it, not by his relationships. As one man described it, "When people would tell me what a good person I was, or what a terrific father I was, I got no real satisfaction out of it. But when I was praised for being competitive and better in doing certain things than other men, it puffed me up. I realized how 'sick' it was, that being seen as a good tennis player affected my self-esteem more than being acknowledged as a good father."

His body is experienced mechanically, like his car. Sexually, his penis is an object that "works" or "doesn't work." He calls it being *objective.*

When the disconnected, impersonal male enters into a relationship with the intimate, inner-directed female, after the initial romantic rush, conflict and pain result as he steers the relationship outside and she tries to bring it closer together. Each person feels pressured and frustrated by these encounters and the difficult attempts to find satisfaction. It is not a happy picture, but it is the principal reason why the best of couples become mired, and why men and women increasingly find a need to relate to one another in cautious, self-protective ways. The pain that occurs in a relationship exists in proportion to a man's disconnection and externalization and a woman's desire for closeness and her focus on inner needs and emotions.

His disconnection and masculinity develop in direct proportion to the suppression of his personal, intimate capacities. The more of "a man" he is, the more this is true. Externalization and internalization cannot exist at the same time because one grows as the other is diminished.

The end point of disconnection is a state of personal oblivion, a "floating away" from the capacity for personal connecting. This is the man who can play with his "toys" for hours on end, but finds it painful to relate personally for even a short period of time. He is anchored by a "long-suffering" wife or female partner who accommodates him and "services" him personally until her pain and frustration become overwhelming.

Until that happens, his focus is on the objective/mechanical/logical and hers is on the subjective/personal/emotional, and this causes conflict and a sense of hopelessness about the relationship. When men and women are on the opposite ends, the conflict, pain, and repression that exist are extreme—and require a maximum of activity, role-bound responsibilities, and distractions such as TV, alcohol, and food, to reduce the tensions.

What Inner Reality Does Defensive Disconnection Create for Him?

The disconnected man's inner experience of the world is a mechanical one. The "meaning" of life is seen as an endless and increasingly complex accumulation of facts, "truths," and objective solutions. The simple and obvious are lost and replaced by a belief that more information and objective analysis will answer all questions and that quest is what makes life meaningful for him.

How Is It Likely to Affect You?

Masculine disconnection is the main source of intense pain and rage in women. It may be experienced as sudden angry outbursts, moodiness, despair, chronic physical symptoms, and the sense of being unloved and abused. Although I am convinced that a man can generate enormous frustration and anger in a woman, *he is being all he can be*. When he is accused of deliberately seeking to hurt and frustrate, he in turn becomes confused and frustrated.

How to Relate to the Effects of His Defensive Disconnection

Keep in mind the following. *Most men don't bond and marry with an intent to hurt. To the extent that they are hurtful, they are as much victims of their conditioning as women.* A relationship must proceed from that awareness.

Understanding the unconscious, defensive behavior of your partner is crucial and can make the difference between a relationship that is destructive and painful, and a relationship that is functional, caring, and has a potential for growth.

Recognizing and acknowledging the inner workings of a man puts into perspective his facade of strength. His is an external strength that exists in proportion to his rigid, brittle, superficial personal being. He is far more emotional than is apparent on the surface and exceedingly vulnerable. Inevitably, victories and power will become hollow and he'll find himself more isolated and depressed as he becomes more successful and powerful.

He is in constant danger of destroying his personal life because of the unconscious drive that propels him increasingly outside of himself and into a negative, isolated, disconnected existence that others interpret as disinterest and a lack of true caring.

Understanding his makeup is a step toward avoiding the draining, endless conflict and crises that result when two people try to change each other.

Most important, knowing the makeup of his deeper self can put an end to the futile illusion of "someone better" out there who will make one happy. The defensive undertow and rhythm between the sexes transform even the most ideal relationship into a similar personal struggle. It is the process that needs to be changed rather than the person.

The Makings of a Successful Man

Whatever is true of men in general is much more applicable to the successful man. Success is not an accident. The process that makes a man a winner in the outside world also makes him a loser in his personal life. The successful man has the most alluring as well as the most undesirable features of the essence of masculinity.

Women married to successful men—physicians, executives, performers, academicians, or athletes—become aware that success is a mixed blessing, with the positive being in the status and external lifestyle symbols, and the negative being in the disconnected features that accompany it and eventually make her feel unneeded, controlled, isolated, and frustrated in her quest for intimacy.

The surgeon who sleeps next to his beeper and who is chronically distracted and preoccupied; the executive who is constantly focused on "the deal"; the professor who is absorbed in his search for truth and solutions and becomes oblivious to those around him; the artist so obsessed with his vision that he is never fully present; and the performer, ever-anxious about his last or next performance, cause women to feel rejected. Relationships with these success-driven men go through the same cycles as other relationships but in more extreme form, beginning with an unusually intense romantic rush and ending with equally intense outpourings of anger, alienation, and total breakdowns in communication.

Successful men are most attractive when they are performing or "doing their thing," and most unappealing when engaging in sustained personal interaction where they tend to become distracted, bored, and self-centered. The closer they come as people (not as achievers) to relating rather than performing, the more the negative aspects impact and erode the positive symbols of success.

The elements that create success develop at the expense of the personal capacities, although his manipulative skills may disguise that fact initially. This is one major cause of the great anger that success-driven men ultimately trigger in their women, who feel betrayed by the initial promise of getting it all only to end up feeling deceived and disappointed.

A woman who chooses a successful man needs to be aware of the pitfalls that accompany her choice. To blame a man for his personal limitations is to blame the traits that attracted her initially.

The Attractive Little Boy Is Father to the Insensitive, Chauvinistic Man

What went wrong? How did the serious, responsible, appealing little boy, the apple of his parents' eyes, and admired by others, grow up to be that *Everyman* accused of being insensitive, cold, critical, and detached?

That is the double-bind and the irony of male conditioning. The very qualities in a little boy that warm our hearts and reassure us that he's "all boy" and destined to be a winner, are the ones that upon extrapolation into adult behavior will defeat him in his personal relationships and cause him to be seen as a sexist or mechanical.

As a boy he is expressing his masculinity outside of an intimate relationship, and it seems attractive. Little boys are most appealing and admired when they are independent, feisty, ambitious, goal directed, fearless, responsible, and active—*not* lazy, emotional, weak, vulnerable, timid, or confused. We are relieved if he has no interest in playing with girls or participating in female-oriented activities, and when nothing intimidates him or causes him to become emotional.

The qualities that make him "all boy" are the same ingredients that will make him an "insensitive" male chauvinist. Even though he seems "nice," "sweet," and considerate as a boy, his "all boy" traits are the same ones that will eventually cause pain and anger in his female partner when he becomes an adult partner in an intertwined personal relationship.

Men are confused and feel betrayed and misunderstood in marriages when behaving as they were taught to from boyhood on, creates such negative responses in adulthood from wives and children. "I don't understand. I don't understand," is the plaint of divorced adult men whose families barely tolerate their presence. He can't see what he did wrong, because in fact, he did it all right.

Prince Charming, or Mr. Rat: The Illusion of the Difference

One woman's lovable "nice guy" is the object of another woman's intense anger and frustration. The woman who hates him now, adored him early on in her relationship when she saw him as her Prince Charming.

The cumulative impact of his defensive core described in this chapter creates the "feeling" parts of a traditional relationship, causing a man to be seen in a much different light in the early stages of a relationship, and in a very negative light at the end. His defensive process impacts and negatively transforms the initial romantic beginnings when he was valued for his symbols of masculinity and not for his capacity for intimacy. The limitations he demonstrates early on tend to be overlooked in the rush of romantic excitement and in the belief that the woman's love will change him and bring out his best qualities. It can't. In fact, pressuring him to be what he is not eventually will do just the opposite.

The impact of process on content is the reason

that the seemingly "perfect couple" eventually experiences the same problems and conflicts as every other couple. This unconscious process is the reason that outsiders looking in on a relationship are puzzled as to why this "perfect couple"—the man and woman who seemed so "nice and loving" at the beginning are now at each others' throats.

The meaning and cure to relationship distress lie in its defensive undertow, which transforms the ideal into the unbearable. The hopeful aspect is that relationship distress can be eliminated if the underlying defensive polarization is dealt with and changed so that both partners can become their best selves and not polarized opposites.

Every man has the potential to be either Prince Charming or Mr. Rat, depending on the process of the relationship. When his limitations are unacknowledged and he is blamed for being what he is and pressured to be what he can't be, his most defensive and distressing behaviors emerge and he becomes Mr. Rat. When the process is balanced and he is not pressured by the defensive needs and insecurities of his polarized opposite, he is free to become his best self.

Who Is "Mr. Macho" and Why Do Women Find Him Offensive?

Just as the attractive boy is father to the chauvinistic adult man, the offensive adult macho is but a heightened version of what "ideal" masculinity is all about and what many women expect and find compelling when they first meet a man.

When traditional unadorned autonomy is expressed to the extreme, it becomes, "I don't need anybody—including you," and "I don't trust anybody because nobody really gives a damn when times get rough."

Dominance and control, become, "No one tells me what to do!" "I know what's right," and "My way or the highway."

Masculine logic and reason in the extreme become acting "cool, calm, and collected" under every circumstance and situation.

Aggression, when fully expressed, makes him a competitor who hates to lose, who will meet any challenge, and whose anger can be explosive and violent.

When his sexuality dominates him, it becomes an obsessive preoccupation with having sex, a tendency to relate to women sexually as objects, with no ability for intimate sharing or communication.

When goal focus is extreme, he will perceive any conversation or activity that doesn't have a concrete purpose as meaningless.

In its full expression, masculine defensiveness is what being a macho pig is all about and what every man has been conditioned to be. Many men and women regard macho behaviors as something distinct and separate, a negative choice some men make rather than simply a heightened degree of a trait that exists in every man.

Why Men "Close Up"

Men will be at their best in a relationship when it involves performance; when they are challenged because a woman's level of self-esteem is consistently high and her identity strong enough that the unspoken message to him is clear: "If you don't value me and give me personal closeness and make that a priority, I'm not staying with you." A display of strength that keeps him perpetually challenged, not by threat but by a woman's inner strength, does wonders to keep men aware and involved.

Men are turned off in relationships in which a woman's low self-esteem and insecurity cause her to seek constant reassurance in ways he can't provide. Slowly, he withdraws until finally, in "self-defense," he shuts down completely. In the end, all men begin to sound the same as they respond, "Leave me alone."

Men "close up" under personal stress, whereas women are more likely to "open up" and reach out under stress. When men are depressed and upset, they tend to become silent and withdrawn and to ignore pleas to seek help or reach out. When women are depressed, they are less reluctant to ask for help or to discuss their problem with a trusted friend.

For this problem to be solved, it needs to be recognized as a two-way dynamic, not a closed-up man with a loving woman. The latter depiction may reassure a woman that it's "his fault," but it guarantees there will be no real change or growth in the relationship.

When left alone to be themselves by a woman

who both recognizes his inherent tendencies and acknowledges the impact of her own needs for reassurance on him, a man will "bounce back" quickly and open himself up at least to the level or capacity he showed during the early romantic phase, when he could relate in an accepting atmosphere of his real self.

Men's Fears and Insecurities

Men's fears and insecurities, though sometimes denied, are reflected indirectly through their obsessive and "insatiable quests"—areas of pursuit where "it's never enough"—and by their rigidities and explosiveness.

Men's competitiveness and their self-hating response when they do poorly reflect their fear of losing and failing.

Men's need to control and their avoidance of situations or environments where they are not in control or are "nobody," reflect their fear of powerlessness.

The need to have a goal or purpose in order to be motivated, and the apparent inability to remain involved without some stated aim, reflect a fear of confronting feelings of not being useful.

The intense anxiety when they are unable to function sexually reflects powerful fears of losing their manliness, or conversely, of being feminine.

Men's avoidance of acknowledging need and the tendency to withdraw when they're troubled reflect an intense fear of being weak, dependent, and vulnerable.

The obsession with logic and facts as the pathway to truth and the distrust of and inability to let go emotionally reflect a fear of losing control of themselves emotionally and of being weak and vulnerable.

Although men may deny these fears and anxieties, the degree to which they are rigid, explosive, compulsive, and predictable in their counteracting responses reflects how frightened and defensive they are underneath, by these "taboo" parts of themselves. The fact that men are prone to act impulsively in self-destructive, life-threatening ways, just to prove they are not afraid, tells us just how powerful these underlying fears really are.

Men's "Blind Spots": How He Distorts His Relationships

When it comes to their personal relationships, men's externalization creates massive blind spots and a vulnerability to gross misjudgment in selecting a partner, dealing with problems, and gauging the state of personal relationships. The latter causes them to be "surprised" and "shocked" when the relationship suddenly ends, or falls into chaos.

Some of the blind spots include:

1. A belief that they will be loved for performing and achieving. The football hero scoring a goal, the young man paying for an expensive night out, the husband working two jobs, the businessman giving his family "the best," all believe that these are sufficient proof of love and will gener-

ate love and loving responses in return. When they don't, he feels betrayed.

2. The belief that the more successful he is the more his wife or partner will be happy and bask in the glory of his accomplishments. He fails to see how the very qualities that produce success may come to alienate those close to him and cause them to resent his success.
3. A belief that his ideas about life are objective truth and can be taught to his children and his wife, who will accept his wisdom with gratitude. His "blind spot," which is an error of projection and "logic," is the belief that what he thinks and believes actually have a reality that exists apart from himself.

   When he discovers that those who are close to him not only don't accept his ideas and act on them, but resent him for imposing them, he is angered and accuses them of being stubborn, naive, or stupid.

   This lack of empathy or inability to recognize that those around him have their own reality and beliefs based on their experiences, is one of his single most powerful barriers to personal relating. This is more of a problem for a successful man whose triumphs convince him that he is "right" about life.

   Those around him may pretend to listen and agree out of intimidation or for manipulative motives. But in the end, he will be embittered by the realization that they are contemptuous of his version of reality.
4. The belief that personal problems can be

solved with impersonal or mechanical solutions represents a massive blind spot. His answer to fears and problems is "willpower," "logic," or "self-control." He gives self-congratulatory pep talks to help others, and alienates those around him. He fails to see his own personal relationship problems resulting from his behavior and how he relates. Instead, he sees them as resulting from "mistakes" he made that have objective, logical remedies.

He believes there are "how to" answers to personal problems. "Do this and you'll be successful," or "Do that and she'll come crawling back to you." The harder and more insistently they push these solutions, the worse matters become.

This blind spot prevents men from learning from their negative personal experiences so they repeat the same damaging patterns over and over.

5. The belief that he is strong and his female partner is fragile, weak, and vulnerable. This reinforces his tendency to feel responsible and guilty when problems arise, and to conceal his thoughts and feelings for fear that it will "crush her."

   Only when the relationship ends does the reality emerge. *He* is the desperate, dependent, fragile one, whereas she is far more resilient and capable of building a new life for herself than he is.

6. Numerous "blind spots" exist in the area of sexuality. Men believe that women will reject them or seek a new lover if they have performance problems. They assume

a woman feels the way a man does about sex and that performance is the priority. When she doesn't reject him for "his impotence," he is grateful and surprised, and sees her as selfless.

One woman explained the reality of her experience this way: "I was actually glad when he became impotent because he started to kiss me more and he became more emotional and tender. Good sex for me is first and foremost being close. If I get that, whether or not he has erections is minor, except for the fact that it bothers him so much. I want to know he needs and loves me. *That* turns me on the most."

7. Sexually, he believes that his dysfunctions are based solely on himself and his "equipment." He perceives his sexual problems as mechanical failures, like broken plumbing, rather than as expressions of what he is feeling and how the relationship is progressing. Thus he feels embarrassed and humiliated by his "failure" and, in desperation, may seek an instant solution or cure. He will fail to find anything but a temporary solution, but his desperate sense of urgency reflects his inability to look meaningfully beyond the surface of the relationship.
8. Men's focus on externals creates a massive blind spot when it comes to being aware of the anger and pain within their partners or their children, and the deterioration or collapse of these relationships. Consequently, when breakdowns do occur, he tends to believe that they were recently

caused. He'll say that "Everything seemed to be going just fine. Oh, there were little things once in a while but they were just minor." This blind spot reflects the depth of his personal alienation from what those around him are actually experiencing.

9. Because of the blind spot in acknowledging and recognizing the pain and alienation of others, there is a strong tendency to minimize or deny altogether, and therefore to ignore, the problems and signs of distress until it is too late. This denial of the long-developing deterioration process then produces the further alienating search for a simplistic solution.
10. He believes that by expressing his ideas more forcefully when he feels he is not being "heard" or listened to, he will be more successful. He is much like an English-speaking person in a foreign country who thinks he can make himself understood by speaking English louder and more slowly. In the process he pushes those close to him away.
11. His need to be right, in control, and validated in his self-image causes a massive blind spot in differentiating when he is being manipulated and when someone truly cares for him. Partially, this creates his "vulnerability" to manipulative women. It results from his tendency to believe that the instant admiration and sexual availability he gets from a woman means that she finds him irresistible. This blind spot may cause serious misjudgments and tragic life consequences.

12. In the face of other people's problems, he believes that his truths about life, and his favorite sayings such as, "Put a smile on your face and you'll feel better," "Practice, practice, practice," or "You can do anything you want—there's no such thing as 'can't'," will help the other person overcome his or her problems. It highlights just how self-involved he really is and how little he knows about those he purports to care about.

The Meaning and Ingredients of His "Mid-Life" Crisis

The alienating impact of his unconscious defensiveness brings him to an inevitable crisis in mid-life. The impact of his disconnection erodes his personal relationships. Furthermore he discovers that his quest for material security and fulfillment through work is an illusion as he grows older and less powerful and as his insecurity increases. No matter how much he has materially, there is never enough.

The moment of truth at mid-life informs him that the negatives far outweigh the positives. The people closest to him, for whom he was supposedly "doing it all," are unhappy with, angry at, or withdraw from him. Put succinctly, one man age forty-seven described it as follows: "I've done my best but it's all turning to garbage and

I can't deny it any longer. The truth is, I have no relationship with my wife and children."

His stereotypical approach to solving his mid-life crisis, such as buying a new sports car, changing his hairstyle, or finding a young girl-friend, mock the depth and severity of the problem. He is trying to ease the pain with the same behavior that created it, and making matters worse because he is destroying the remaining vestiges of caring and concern from those close to him through his ineffective alienating solutions.

Nevertheless, his mid-life crisis is a composite of a whole series of end points that emerge predictably from a lifetime of external, impersonal pursuits that have taken him totally away from his personal self.

The specific ingredients that comprise the crisis include:

1. A sense of inner deadness. There is little in life that can make him feel excited and optimistic.
2. Repetitive conflicts and fights with his wife that never get solved and that make him feel hopeless and frustrated. He has given up believing that things will change or that she will ever understand him.
3. A declining or even nonexistent sexual interest in his partner. What was once a source of pleasure and anticipation has become a cause for distress and avoidance. "I can't please her and I'm not getting anything from this either," he realizes.
4. An awareness that his quest for financial security is endless. Even if he could retire,

he seems to have lost the capacity to function and enjoy life without working.

5. The awareness that his wife is always unhappy, tired, or complaining of feeling ill. Even when it is not said directly, it is implied that he is to blame. *He* has made her unhappy.
6. An absence of closeness with his own children who have disappointed him. "They only talk to me when they want money," is a commonly expressed feeling.

   He has alienated them by forcing his values on them, which they have rejected. "They didn't turn out as I'd hoped," is the way many men express their disappointment. In addition, there is resentment because the children seem to be closer to their mother and because they seem ungrateful about his contributions.
7. A sense of overall failure in obtaining the personal goals and dreams that he'd hoped to achieve by mid-life. Life isn't turning out anywhere near what it was supposed to.
8. The feeling that he betrayed himself because he never really did it "his way" and that at mid-life it's "now or never," if he's ever going to risk being "totally himself."
9. A sense of hopelessness because the ideals and values he based his life on have revealed themselves to be false. He has become a "bottom liner," cynically putting a priority on his own self-interests and manipulating those in his professional life whom he pretends to care about.
10. A feeling that his life increasingly has

become a series of pressures and responsibilities. Instead of becoming easier, life has become more difficult. There is no balancing element to justify continuing the struggle.

11. A growing sense that his needs and feelings don't really matter to those close to him. He is only there to provide for them. They seem disinterested in him, his needs, his feelings, and he is a stranger to them.
12. Increasing fantasies about other women and what it would be like to give in to sexual abandon.
13. Weekends, holidays, vacations, and special occasions that he has come to dread because they are more stressful than going to work. This too makes the idea of a happy retirement an illusion because it would mean giving up the major means of escape from his personal problems.
14. A belief that from mid-life on, unless he makes a change, things will only get worse.

Finally, a growing impatience and anger lurk constantly just below the surface and he can't stand himself any more than others can. He feels compelled to begin again.

Men at Their Best

His externalization means that he will be at his best and most comfortable as a *doer*, providing materially, being protective, taking responsibility and control, working toward goals, confronting external challenges, and being someone others can lean on for support.

These are the ways traditional men love. To have those aspects discounted because of his limitations in personal relating would be the same as a man criticizing a woman because she is not ambitious, successful, and aggressive enough in her career, even though she is a giving and loving partner in their personal interaction.

Men give differently than women. Men show love in line with their development: they do what they can do, they give as best they can.

The tragedy is that the ways men have been taught to give and love are not experienced as such by their partners. Too often, they are discounted as being self-centered and hurtful, because only their negative traits are responded to.

Boys and young men are applauded for their accomplishments. They are encouraged to be loving but not at the expense of competitive drive and achievement. Emphasis is on performance. Women in relationships often believe that men choose to be hurtful or self-absorbed. In fact, many men avoid being overly demonstrative because of the negative responses they received in early childhood whenever they were any less than "all boy."

To diminish the way men give and love is to reject them for being who they are. A woman who does this belies the notion that she loves her partner and has a greater capacity for closeness than he does. To love him is to love him for who and what he is, and to acknowledge and recognize that objectively. To love him is to be understanding of what he may be incapable of giving.

3

He Says: What Men in Relationships Say to Themselves but not Always to Their Partners

The tendency to "close up" is already present in men because of boyhood modeling. His silent father was an equation of manliness, with action, not words. As a boy his role models in films and comics kept their own counsel. When they spoke, it was important.

One man described still being able to hear the voice of his father admonishing, "Talk is cheap," "You sound like a gossipy woman," or "Silence is golden," when he "talked too much." He reflected: "When I would try and talk to Dad, I could see his eyes glaze over. He'd look bored and distracted. Or he would start to lecture me about what I was saying before he heard me out.

"I never learned to listen because I was never listened to myself. What we did 'talk about' were impersonal or objective things where it was a matter of having information and correct answers. I never learned to discuss things without a purpose or a point to justify it."

Therefore, on the one hand, when men close up in personal relationships, some of it is natural masculine defensive self-protection. Some of his continuing to "not open up," however, is a result of what he experiences in the relationship and is something he might have tried to communicate. Giving up on making himself heard or understood, he gradually does what traditional men do. His conversation becomes increasingly limited or perhaps he stops talking personally altogether.

Stephen, forty-three years old, described his experience in relationships. "Women don't really want to know what I feel, like they seem to think they do," he said. "Initially, when I believed them about that, I often found that later I regretted it. Despite assurances that it was safe to risk and disclose what I felt, what I said was often judged 'not nice,' distancing, or unloving. When I revealed my conflicts and resistances in the relationship, I usually received an angry or tearful response with punishing by-products like her getting cold, withdrawn, or suggesting that we end the relationship. I guess I learned that 'opening up' was dangerous and rarely worth it."

Often men are surprised by the extreme reaction they get to something they thought was an innocuous, nonthreatening comment, or even a tongue-in-cheek, joking remark. Or what he believed to be an innocent attempt to be honest, or when he was "just being myself," it was interpreted as being critical and mean. Because most men have an exaggerated sense of their ability to hurt or disappoint their partner "if she really knew me," they often tend to feel guilty, become increasingly self-conscious, and withdraw. "You can't say that to a woman," is something men tell one another when recounting these experiences. It leads to a conditioning in which fewer honest feelings are communicated.

For these and many other reasons, important relationship reactions and responses of men remain unsaid or are communicated inadequately. The following are representative of some of these unspoken, inner relationship experiences of men.

About Sharing Feelings

The following quotes are composites of what I have been told by many men.

"I've given up trying to tell a woman I'm involved with how I feel. She only really listens when I say 'nice' or 'loving' things. Whenever I try to communicate anything else, I can feel her getting defensive and upset."

"If I want to avoid a battle, lingering bad feelings, and all the back-and-forth dancing to reassure her that I really want to be with her, and that what I said didn't mean I didn't love her it's best I confine myself to the positive and neutral. Since that gets empty and repetitive, I find myself having less and less to say."

"She may not like the fact that I'm quiet, but I can justify that to her. At least I don't get into bottomless discussions about what I 'really meant' and how I 'really feel' about us that only make me feel worse the longer they go on."

"When I go away on business for a few days, and she asks if I missed her, and I don't answer in just the right way because I'm preoccupied, worried, or because I actually feel that I work better when I don't have to worry about her on a trip, she reacts with statements such as, 'Maybe you don't want to be with me any longer.' Then I have to explain and reassure her that it doesn't mean I don't care about her."

What He Needs in Order to Open Up

Women who want men to reveal themselves need to be aware of their part in generating his reluctance to doing so. Men feel helpless and hopeless explaining themselves in the face of accusations that they are unloving, rejecting, insensitive, or even cruel.

Most men would reveal themselves more if their words were heard as they intended them and not as interpreted by their partner. Accused of being hostile, insensitive, sexist, rejecting, or self-centered and getting a reaction of tears or threats to end the relationship assures men's "closing up."

About Being Close

"How can I be close to a woman when she doesn't acknowledge her equal part in and responsibility for the problems we have? How can

I get close to someone who makes me the 'bad guy,' and sees herself as loving and blameless?"

"How can I feel close to someone who continually tells me about my deficiencies as a caring or loving person? I couldn't be as limited and bad at love as I'm portrayed to be, or if I really am, my logical mind asks why would she even want to get close anyway and how could she really love *me* as she says that she does?"

An experienced bachelor who describes himself as having been around the relationship track many times reflected, "In all my years in and out of relationships with educated, sophisticated, professional women I have *rarely* been with a woman who, on a regular basis, could recognize and acknowledge how her reactions and behavior affected me and contributed to the responses and behaviors of mine that bothered her.

"It seems almost congenital, it's so consistent, this inability to see herself as an equal ingredient in the overall chemistry and dynamic of our relationship.

"In relationships, women seem to think that everything loving originates in them, and everything hurtful originates in the man. When I'm with a woman who sees herself as an equal ingredient, I start to feel close and act close, and I love it."

What He Needs in Order to Get Close

Many men express frustration over how an insensitive action or word may be amplified, whereas the caring and loving responses are minimized or seen as trivial or even insincere. Feeling themselves flawed, rejected, or misunderstood, they maintain an emotional distance, which disguises frustration and anger.

Although men's objective or impersonal style can make them seem selfish and hurtful, men in relationships see themselves as trying hard to be close, and feeling that they would respond more favorably if that was acknowledged; they also feel that their resistance to being close (when it appears) may be a legitimate reaction to frustration over a woman's unwillingness to "share the blame."

About Understanding Women

"Are women crazy, or do I, without knowing exactly how, somehow make them as irrational and volatile as they seem to become after we get involved? They're rarely like that until after we get 'serious.' "

Although women perceive in men a cold and selfish quality, many men are bewildered by the extreme shifts in a woman's mood for which they are often blamed.

Things seem to become most irrational when men try to be logical in the face of an emotional outburst. She will suddenly and "for no apparent reason" become more hostile or start to cry. When asked why, she'll answer in ways that make no sense to him.

A seasoned book publishing executive recounted the "nightmare" of "irrationality" that occurred in the last few years of his marriage. "I got into a running argument that finally blew my 'logical' mind," he told me. "I'd play golf on Saturday afternoon—my favorite and only recreation on my only full day off.

"I'd arrive home around 6:30. For some reason unknown to me, my wife thought that I should be home by 6:00. I'd ask her, 'Why? What's the difference? What's going on that requires my presence here at 6:00?' She wouldn't answer. She'd just get angrier. I couldn't give in to her without some sensible explanation and cater to her irrationality; but I couldn't get an explanation." Similar kinds of unresolvable arguments led him to believe, as some men do, that women are possessed. "She needed exorcism, not therapy," he remarked.

What He Needs in Order to Understand a Woman

Men's logic is often only logical to them, and is perceived as a weapon used to avoid emotions in the relationship. Women who want to relate to men's reality, however, need to realize how a woman's emotional response, in the midst of an argument, triggers an aggressive desperation in him, particularly when he feels that he can't "get through" the emotional reactions he triggers. Men are conditioned to be analytic problem solvers, not empathic, emotional partners, and they tend to overreact and become defensive if they can't use reason. Being critical of his "coldness" and need to analyze also contributes to an extreme breakdown of communication.

About Putting Women Down

"I don't feel or intend to be critical of a woman, even though I hear, regularly, that I am. I'm accused of being patronizing, sarcastic, or of putting her down, and it bewilders me. Nor do I want to control a woman or use her, but I hear that a lot too.

"If I seem to be that way, I wish I could get specific examples, instead of blame me for my attitude or tone. I honestly have no clue sometimes exactly what women are referring to, and often I can't get a straight answer though I really want to know.

"The funny thing is, I hear that criticism most when I see myself trying to be helpful and supportive—but it doesn't seem to come through. I think I'm going one way and find out that I'm seen as going the opposite way."

For example, one man gave up trying to relate to a woman he was strongly attracted to when he found himself accused of being patronizing when he "instinctively" opened the car door for her, and carried her food tray to the table at a buffet where they were having brunch.

Jim, a thirty-four-year-old single man, initially was very drawn to Kristin. Because they were both psychotherapists, he presumed that he could be direct and unself-conscious in expressing himself around her and that if she had a problem about anything he did or said, he felt confident that she would simply tell him and they could work out any differences.

He was shocked to the point of feeling he had to end the relationship when, after six months of dating, during which he felt the relationship was progressing well, and that he had been loving to her, she presented him with a long list of ways in which she felt he had been "critical" of her.

Another man, back from a second honeymoon vacation in Mexico, which he hoped would bring romance and passion back to a relationship that had become distant and cold, found that his efforts to be thoughtful and affectionate had failed. His wife told him how painful the trip had been because she felt he had been cutting her off in the middle of her sentences around two other couples they socialized with, and because he seemed bored by her conversation.

Although he could acknowledge his bad habit of dominating conversations, he felt defeated, hearing that his efforts to be loving had made no impact, and only his negative responses were remembered.

How to Help Him Understand How His Actions Tend to "Put Women Down"

Women can understand men's frustration in this area by reflecting on a counterpart experience, which is the "woman who loves too much." A woman in that situation is bewildered and angered when her expressions of love trigger only coldness, selfishness, and exploitation in response. She sees herself giving love, but the man is not experiencing it as love and so his response is cold. However, she cannot see how her efforts at loving are actually alienating, just as men can't understand what they do to trigger a woman's anger when they believe they are being supportive and loving.

Women who feel abused or criticized by a man and who want to understand why, will begin to do so if they can accept that often he doesn't intend to be that way. In fact, he may see himself as doing just the opposite. It is safe to say that in marriage or committed relationships, controlling, critical, or cold responses from men often are nothing personal. Communicating her reactions, and also considering the possibility that she is overly sensitive to whatever smacks of criticism from a man, would be a constructive starting point.

About Being Honest

"Sure I lie to the woman I'm involved with. When I've risked being fully honest with my thoughts or feelings, unless they were 'nice' or neutral, I've gotten distressing reactions. It's not worth it," was a typical response from men discussing the issue of honesty in relationships.

In committed relationships, because intimate, close relating is not easy or comfortable, men may have feelings and thoughts that are "not nice," or can be easily misunderstood or seem to be more negative than intended. When his wife is indecisive, he may become irritated and impatient because his tendency is to act or decide quickly. When she "pressures" for a reassuring hug, kiss, or other expression of love, he may feel uncomfortable because affectionate behavior is not his style. In bed, he may fantasize about other women because he has been sexually conditioned on fantasy. These behaviors are byproducts of an entrenched socialized totality, out of which emerges the good as well as the bad in his personality. They are responses not meant personally.

He is in a double-bind. If he conveys his true feelings, he is likely to be misunderstood and defensively reacted to and seen as hurtful. He can soon become the dishonest male, hiding the negative thoughts, experiences, and feelings that he may come to deny, even to himself.

What He Needs in Order to Risk Being Fully Honest

Because women convey a strong need for emotional security and love, so much of what a man thinks or feels becomes unspeakable, lest he "hurt" her and irreparably damage the relationship. "I'll never make her understand me, so I might as well say nothing at all," is how one man expressed it.

Particularly at the beginning of a relationship, conflict is normal. How this conflict is managed and how responsibility for it is taken will separate positive from destructive relationships. Women who become tearful and/or accusing of the male and feed on his tendency to feel guilty and responsible when he reveals himself in a real effort to communicate, will win short-term battles but contribute to the destruction of a relationship as he learns to withhold honest expressions of himself.

The man who is truly honest will inevitably say and do things that seem threatening to his partner, but they are not meant that way. Acceptance of what he shares, reacting to them not as personal attacks but as expressions of who and what he is, will begin a cycle of trust and openness that will ultimately generate the kind of love and intimacy that is rooted in honesty.

About Selfless Women

"Women are wonderful at giving you what you don't want or need and ignoring, discounting, or resisting what is important to you. In the former, they expect you to respond with delight anyway, and in the latter, they think you're awful for feeling angry and disappointed?" Eric, age thirty-seven and married, talked about his experience. He described what happened when he didn't respond appreciatively to a gift his wife bought that he didn't like. "She said I was killing her enthusiasm and feelings of love and that she'd never go out of her way to be thoughtful again. That's not how I want it," he said.

"I love having thoughtful, caring things done that I've asked for, or made known are important to me. Too often, however, when I am direct in what I want, like the time I was watching a ball game and asked her to make me a sandwich, the response is a resentful one such as 'I'm not your housekeeper.' "

Michael described his struggle with his live-in partner. "She greets me at the door after work with lots of hugs and kisses, which I have a hard time responding to when I first come home because I'm so damned wired and preoccupied. I know she's hurt if I don't act happy and delighted, and I don't know what to do. It sounds chauvinistic, but if she wants to love me, give me what I can handle, or don't give me anything so at least I won't feel guilty and pressured."

Self-centered love means giving something to someone that is designed primarily to benefit and satisfy the giver, while appearing to benefit the other person. Men are guilty of that when they rationalize their workaholism as something they're doing for the family, or when they give advice or try to be helpful in insensitive ways and expect a grateful reaction. Women who love men in ways that satisfy primarily their own needs are giving "self-centered love" as well.

One man described his experience. "On my fortieth birthday, my wife 'gave me' a surprise party. Since we've been together eight years, she must know that not only don't I like birthday parties, but I was depressed about turning forty. I was questioning where I was going, my friendships, and almost everything. It was the worst time to give me a party. In fact, I asked her not to.

"Instead, she went all out with catered food my already bloated body didn't need and invited many people I didn't feel particularly good about. During the course of the party, she kept coming over and telling me to smile and not be a 'party pooper.' It was agony.

"Then came time for the opening of gifts. She told everybody to bring gag gifts. Most brought something alluding to my being over the hill sexually. I couldn't get with the humor.

"After the party, she was angry and hurt. Her phrase, 'At least you could have tried to be nice,' still rings in my ears. I knew then why I'd been having a problem being loving with her. She was 'loving me' her way. It had nothing to do with how I felt, what I needed, and who I was.

"She was really convinced I was selfish and negative and I couldn't get her to see how she affected me. I was the one who couldn't accept or give love, according to her."

What He Needs in Order to Appreciate Being Loved

The result of getting "narcissistic love" is a feeling of being oppressed and depressed at the inability to be happy in a relationship that is supposed to feel good but doesn't. Until this cycle is broken and women "give" according to a man's reality and experience, neither women nor men will be able to experience the man's loving potential. His energy will be tied up in conflict and self-hatred over his negative response to "love" that doesn't relate to who he is and therefore doesn't feel good to him.

Women desiring to achieve genuine love and intimacy need to abandon all of their preconceptions about what men need and what makes men feel good. Then women need patience, because most men find it difficult to define exactly what they really do need. They have not been taught to express their needs clearly, and thus share responsibility for the creation of their dilemma.

As the relationship progresses, women need to check with the man to determine whether it is something they want, before they go ahead and give it. Then genuine loving would mean accepting what he says, without negative judgments.

For the sake of the relationship, it is better to do nothing for a man than to do something that is intended to be loving, and which the man is then expected to respond to positively.

About Giving Her Emotional Security

"No matter how much I tell her I am committed and love her, it's never enough. One 'wrong' or 'insensitive' remark negates a hundred that are positive and reassuring.

"Out of nowhere, she will ask, 'Do you still love me?' or 'Do you love me as much as ever?' This always catches me off guard. When I don't respond well because I am affected by the pressure and suddenness of her question, she takes it as a rejection.

"She'll tell me I never loved her in the first place, which is not true. Why on earth would I be with her if I didn't love her in the first place? If she thinks I'm only with her because I'm afraid to be alone, or because I'm using her, then she couldn't think very much of me.

"After a number of those episodes of her acting insecure, needy, and challenging my feelings and intentions, I do become withdrawn and defensive. Doubts do come in because her sensitivity takes away from the pleasure of being together and creates a relentless pressure to always prove my love."

Another man voiced a similar inner experience. "The pressure of proving my love," he said, "is grinding me down and causing me to wonder whether my love for her is real, and whether I should even be here."

What He Needs in Order to Be Emotionally Supportive

Because men express love differently from women, women often disbelieve that what a man does to show love is real. At the same time, demonstrations of verbal and physical affection are more difficult. In his spontaneous reactions, unwittingly he may express things that seem rejecting because of his difficulty in expressing that part of himself. But he does not intend to be insensitive or hurtful. Both men and women have areas of self-expression that have been blocked.

A man hears from his partner, "My feelings don't go like yours—on again, off again. Even when you try and show me your love, it doesn't feel like love. Sometimes when you're with me, it doesn't feel like you're even here."

When men hear these kinds of statements, they can do nothing except stand by helplessly and resentfully because from their vantage point these accusations seem unfair and unwarranted. Confusion, anger, and frustration build in them over time as a result of having their loving feelings doubted or construed negatively.

About His Not Being Good Enough

"In intimate relationships, once I commit myself," one man told me, "it becomes 'open season' for criticism, and showing me how inadequate I am as a partner, a father, a lover, and a husband. I come to feel that I'm doing well if she doesn't look unhappy and I'm not being told I'm uninvolved, self-centered, or unfeeling."

Reflecting on family outings, Jerry, a divorced man in his forties, remembered, "When we'd be with the children on weekends, nothing I did was quite right. Either I was talking too much or I was too quiet. Or, I was told I was interacting with the kids and ignoring my wife, or I wasn't interacting enough with them and was putting all the responsibility for the children on her, and having selfishly fun time. Or it was pointed out to me that I was preoccupied and thinking about work and only going through the motions because I didn't really want to be there."

What He Needs in Order to Feel Good About Himself in the Relationship

Criticisms that do not take into account his inner experience and reality make social and family experiences unpleasant and stressful. Men tend to withhold their reactions to criticism because it feeds on their self-doubts about whether they really can love and promotes the self-conscious, negative, and detached behaviors and discontent that their conditioning has already made them prone to do.

Men's socialization has not promoted the development of intimate behaviors. However, acceptance of who and what they are, and the realization that they do express love in ways they know how to, bring out their best. Confrontations about their inadequacies in intimacy and questioning their sincerity or caring eventually will produce withdrawal and feelings of futility.

About Euphoric Beginnings and Disastrous Endings

"Don't first adore me; telling me how wonderful I am for the wrong reasons, then become angry and hateful toward me later on for the wrong reasons, again because I wasn't who you thought I was or who you wanted me to be in the first place. And through it all, you never related to me as I am," was the reflection of an unmarried man who had experienced many "hot" beginnings and painful endings.

A European actor, famed for engendering powerful romantic feelings in women, summarized a lifetime of such experiences. Talking about relationships, he described how initially women perceived him as sweet and gentle, then always came to see him as a monstrous egotist. He conceded that he'd rather be less loved and more respected for what he really was.*

The man about whom a woman speaks bitterly and with blaming rage at the end of the relationship, is essentially the same man she described as wonderful, special, and "different from other men" at the beginning. As a therapist for many men over the years, I can testify how slowly real change actually occurs in men.

The man, as he really is, is rarely the object of a woman's romantic passion initially. What many women fall in love with in the beginning is equivalent in objectivity to a man's falling in love with a beautiful face or body.

Consequently, few women ever recognize and relate to the actual qualities and inner reality of most men, who are not as wonderful as they are initially perceived, nor as bad and insensitive as they are described to be at the end. A real relationship has never taken place.

I believe that men are in part unconsciously reluctant to commit to relationships because they sense the dangers and inevitable progression and deterioration caused by initial romantic infatuation. The joys of being placed on a pedestal are seductively powerful but hazardous, because men can't live up to what women see in them at the beginning.

Men's egos crave and therefore are vulnerable to the initial adoring feedback they get. They pay the price by carrying a burden of responsi-

---

*Brad Darrach, "Marcello Mastroianni," *People* (December 17, 1987), p. 105.

bility for being someone they're not and they end up being sources of disappointment, anger, and feelings of betrayal in their partner.

One man summarized his effort to be seen as he saw himself. "After the honeymoon period, I tried to get Linda to acknowledge and appreciate me as I was, without disenchanting her and turning her off. I failed miserably. Whenever I'd say to her, 'But this is who I am,' during an argument, she'd think I was being sarcastic or deliberately hurtful.

"Something is seriously wrong with so-called love relationships where you're wildly inflated initially, then wind up being seen as the scum of the earth at the end. That, more than anything else, tells me how screwed up most relationships are and that is what I'm most fearful of in committing myself. The irony is that most women really believe they want to get to know a man as he really is."

What He Needs in Order to Maintain the Momentum of Romantic Beginnings

When a man says, "This is who I am," believe him; accept it as an important communication and ask yourself whether you can love him based on how he knows himself to be.

Men who inspire intense romantic feelings in women initially, rarely have what women hope for to follow through toward a romantic development of closeness and intimacy. Don't expect that and don't be disappointed when it doesn't happen. Intimacy can't occur without difficult transition periods, during which his ways of relating are seen, accepted, and worked on.

About Who's Using Whom?

"Let's not call this marriage a relationship. A husband is not a person, he is a responsibility and a performance object," one man said.

When men get in touch with their real feelings and with what's going on in their marriage, they often have the same sense of being used as "objects" as their wives, who angrily come to regard themselves as appliances or "service stations." He will describe feeling like "a wallet," or "the garbage man," because providing and doing the "dirty tasks" is how he's related to.

Men are particularly slow to recognize when they are being used in relationships because they learn to expect that treatment as a result of their boyhood experiences.

As young athletes, for example, when their performance deteriorates, so does their right to compete and be involved. However, in most marriages the love of a wife for her husband is as contingent on his role, performance, and "use," as is the love of a chauvinist husband for "his woman."

What He Needs in Order to Relate Person-to-Person, not Object-to-Object

A more productive starting point for improving the quality of relationships, for both sexes, would be to acknowledge the use of the other. Initially men are evaluated not for how they are as people, but for their potential as "husbands," based on careers, education, finances, and family background. For either sex to see itself as being used without acknowledging its own motives guarantees the deterioration of the relationship via self-righteous feelings of being exploited.

In traditional relationships men use women and women use men. If they were mainly friends, relating person-to-person, relationships would not disintegrate or deteriorate as they do. Matters could be discussed, renegotiated, resolved, and improved. Male-female relationships would be stable and "predictable." The reality, however, is that conflict is rarely resolved in positive, productive ways because of the denial and unconscious defensiveness that characterize the object-to-object, mutual using aspects of relationships. Consequently, when the person behind the object emerges, trouble arises and the relationship tends to deteriorate rather than solidify.

Listen to the comments of a number of men:

"When I hear the word 'husband,' I tighten up. I don't think it's because I'm afraid of commitment. It's that being a husband is a job—a role with never-ending 'shoulds.' A husband is 'supposed to be' all sorts of great things, many of which I know I'm not very good at. So it's a setup because in the end I'll be seen as the 'lousy husband.' "

Commented another, "Now I know what women meant when they said, 'I need a wife—I don't want to be a wife.' That's how I feel. I don't want to be a husband. I need a husband. I feel used for what I can do, and never loved for who I am."

It was cogently put by a young man considering marriage: "I don't mind being an object if she'll acknowledge that's what I am to her, and not holier-than-thou me about how loving she is and how afraid to love or be loved I am.

"Why not begin with some honesty about how we need each other for our roles and negotiate based on that initial reality? At least then I won't be solely the one accused. Objects don't get close. Hopefully, people can."

About Being Heard

"Who's not listening to whom? I don't feel heard either," was the frustrated response of a number of men whom I interviewed.

When men try to make their motives or interpretations of things understood, too often it sounds to women like justification or a way to rationalize a lack of involvement. "When I provide information or state my opinion, I notice my wife getting bored or distracted," indicated one man. "I feel she's not interested."

"When I tell her she's not listening, she answers, 'I don't believe you really want to talk to me—or about us, anyway. I could be just about anybody. So why should I pay attention?' " His feelings of not being listened to is discounted or justified by the woman, because she feels that his talk is too impersonal or not heartfelt.

What He Needs in Order to Learn to Listen and to Feel Heard

When men speak analytically or objectively, women react badly to what they see as a lack of emotion and caring. Although it may seem that way to her, he experiences himself as trying to be communicative. It is how he has learned to communicate. If what he says is heard and accepted as being a well-intentioned effort at communication, the best of his loving potential can emerge because he feels heard—which is the cornerstone to feeling assured that talking is useful.

About Fragile Women and Destructive Men

"I don't want that kind of power over a woman—to feel that I can destroy her with a wrong word or misbehavior. I don't want that vulnerable and helpless feeling I get from some women that makes me feel a lot more powerful with her than I want to be."

When a woman is unhappy, many men feel that it's because of something they did or said. When the sex is bad, he failed to "turn her on." When he talks or acts spontaneously and discovers that he said or did something hurtful, and "spoiled" the day, he is given a "power" to be "destructive," which is a negative burden. Men respond best to women who will engage in direct give-and-take without responses that make him feel guilty of being cruel and insensitive. The feeling that he will have that effect, I believe, is a significant element in diminishing a man's desire to communicate.

What He Needs in Order to Relate to Women Realistically

Women are far stronger than men think they are, and, similarly, men are far more vulnerable and fragile than they seem to be. At the end of the relationship, the "fragile" woman often fares better in her new life than the "invulnerable" man.

The perceptual distortions that cause the sexes to misperceive their partner—with women frequently feeling controlled and abused and men feeling responsible, guilty, and hurtful prevents the relationship from becoming a friendship of equal responsibility.

It has been an unfortunate reality of male/female polarization, that women don't demonstrate and maintain their power, autonomy, and assertiveness until they are ready to end a relationship, and men don't experience their vulnerability, dependency, and fear until they are abandoned.

Both sexes have areas of power and of helplessness in relationships. A loving relationship recognizes the vulnerability and strength of each so that neither party ends up feeling controlled, manipulated, or abused.

About Being Nice

"I know she wants things to be 'nice,' but 'nice' all the time irritates and bores me. It feels phony and there's always that pressure on me to be nice in return if she's always that way. I don't feel that way, so it adds insult to injury. I'm the bad guy for not feeling in a way that I see as phony and deadening.

"I like women better and I trust them more," said one man, "if they are direct and 'not nice.' 'Nice' women always make me feel guilty and inadequate, which makes me feel manipulated.

"I want to shake 'nice' women and say 'stop it! This is boring and dead and unreal. One day you'll turn on me and give it to me with both barrels and you'll say it's my fault because I didn't know how to be nice. If you love me, then stop being so damn nice and show me your other side.' "

A man who had experienced a number of failed romances remarked, "In my relationships, the 'nicer' the woman was at the beginning, the angrier she was in the end. I guess I injured her sensibilities. Also, while you're involved with them, the really "nice" women seem always tired, sick, or they can't make decisions. I guess they're sitting on a lot of negative feelings that they deny.

"Sex with a 'nice' woman is not fulfilling either. I mean, the kind where the woman ends up saying, 'That was very nice!' or 'Wasn't that nice?' and you know she hardly got anything out of it. She just wants to be nice."

What He Needs in Order to Be Consistently "Nice"

The problem with trying to keep a relationship at a "nice" level is that invariably men feel like the spoiler because they can't maintain the same level of "niceness" as women, who are more comfortable with "nice" than with confrontation. When he's asked, "Why can't you at least try and be nice?" his inner reaction is to feel chastised and hopeless about ever getting certain feelings and conflicts out in the open.

I believe "nice" on a constant basis is defensive denial. A man who is not "nice" is not being uncaring or "not trying." A woman who wants to create a genuine state of "niceness" needs to be comfortable with accepting the existence of the "not nice" feelings in the man, in herself, and in the relationship, so that conflict can be resolved and angry feelings released, and true "niceness" expressed.

About Being Supportive

"When a woman tells me her plans or dreams and I don't respond immediately with great enthusiasm, she thinks that I'm really down on her. Skeptical, maybe. But that's the way I am about all 'exciting ideas,' including my own that are still in the initial stages.

"A woman will announce a dream, such as opening a shop, or being an artist, and I'm supposed to help make it happen or share her excitement. If I don't, it means that I'm against her.

"I can't always be a woman's cheerleader, nor do I want to be pressured to say, 'It's great,' when I can see the potential obstacles and disappointments. If I bring them up, I'm accused of 'raining on her parade,' or being unsupportive. If I nod and hold my tongue, I'm called 'unenthusiastic.' "

One man described his experience. "My wife told me she was going to take writing classes, buy a word processor, and write children's books and magazine articles to supplement our income. I thought to myself, 'Does she know what's involved in breaking into publishing and how long it takes to get good enough at it to make money?' Yes, I had serious doubts and some anger because we needed extra income, but I chose to react in a neutral way.

"Bam! Before I knew it, she was dropping her plans to go back to school and I was guilty of quashing her ambition. She said I didn't want her to do it. I really felt manipulated and now I tell her I don't want to hear her plans until she's already acted on them."

Another man commented, "I'm pleased if she's pleased, but I resent the pressure to be excited in order to reassure her that I'm not being negative or responsible for helping her maintain her enthusiasm."

What He Needs in Order to Become Supportive

Genuine support requires honest input, not just encouragement and enthusiasm. Men become encouraging and enthusiastic if they feel they can discuss "the realities" as they see them.

To the extent that a man is hard on himself, and critical of others, he will tend to focus more on the down sides than on the possibilities of a new situation. Realizing that, women should either keep cherished plans to themselves until they're launched or not request input from their partner.

If a woman can accept a man's "critical" feedback without attributing damaging motives to him, she is then much more likely to gain his respect and enthusiastic support.

Conclusion

Men experience things differently than women. The surest way to "open up" a man is to listen without judgment, and without negative emotional reactions to what he says. Every hurt response or harsh judgment about the sensitivity, loving capacity, or caring of a man will only cause him to become wary, distrustful, and to close up. He may not even be aware that he is withdrawing. Similarly, he will open up not by request, but by an understanding attitude that allows him to express his inner feelings without his partner reacting as if these opinions are damaging and destructive.

4

Women Ask Why: Common and Not-So-Common Questions About Men

Judy and Jim loved each other but couldn't have a dialogue about anything personal without triggering each other's anger and frustration. Jim would talk about having to save more money and Judy would call him "neurotically frugal" or "cheap like your father." Jim would explode: "You don't understand what my concerns about money and the future are, do you? You have this picture of the world that lets you feel that somehow we don't have to worry about tomorrow. Well, I don't see life that way. I always need to feel I'm prepared for the worst-case scenario."

Or, while shopping at the mall, Jim's eyes might move in the direction of an attractive girl, and he might comment about her "sexy walk." Judy would feel hurt and Jim would try to explain that looking at girls was simply a way to pass time because shopping was dull and that looking had nothing to do with his feelings about Judy.

Jim and Judy loved each other, but the strain caused by these misunderstandings was beginning to make them doubt whether they should stay together. Why had things seemed so perfect, with such easy communication when they first met, and why was it becoming increasingly difficult to talk? And why, even though both of them were sophisticated and educated, did they misinterpret each other's seemingly innocent statements?

When men and women confuse and infuriate each other, often it is because they speak a different language, even as they use the same words and think they are being clear and obvious. Or, when in the early romantic phase, they believe that they understand each other so completely that they don't even need to use words, it becomes obvious in the final phase of the relationship when this same couple can barely manage a few sentences without triggering angry and painful responses that they really don't understand each other.

There is much to understand on both sides, without blame or prejudgment, about the filtering and translating process of each sex and the inner reality and meaning each brings to the same words.

It seems that because women in relationships almost always come to see themselves as treated insensitively by self-centered men, they become resistant to hearing and understanding the reality of men who trigger their pain and disappointment. Feeling wounded, they expect men to change unilaterally, and real change in the relationship becomes impossible.

In these chapters I am addressing the woman who can acknowledge that men actually want to relate to women with sensitivity and compassion and do not intend to be the "selfish" and "abusive" individuals they are often portrayed as; and that they have an equally valid story to tell of an inner experience of frustration and helplessness in the face of the misunderstandings and arguments with the women they love.

By answering the "whys" of the male experience and the reasons behind men's response, this chapter should provide guidelines to allow a woman in a relationship to respond in sync with the man's experience and reality.

The destruction of intimate man/woman communication occurs as a result of several powerful unconscious elements.

First, there are opposing internal "definitions" of loving behavior that result from different early experiences. Thus what one sex learns is an expression of love is not viewed that way by the other sex. The intense focus and emphasis on a new relationship and the desire for increasing closeness that women feel are part of the natural loving process, for example, may not feel that way to men, who experience it as pressure; just as the "doing for" and taking responsibility and initiative that men believe are an expression of their love may not feel that way to the women receiving it.

In the face of contradictory perceptions, men eventually feel smothered, engulfed, and needing to pull away from what women believe are their expressions of loving, whereas women feel they are being distanced, rejected, controlled, and unloved by the man who is only trying to create protective boundaries. Then both may feel hurt and angry at the response they get for giving love, but not getting it back.

Then there is the conviction on both sides that the other person could respond differently if he or she only wanted to. There is a denial in both sexes of the ways they trigger and promote the distressing and defensive response that they accuse the other sex of intentionally expressing to be hurtful.

In order to understand his experience and his actions, women need to understand the effects of his masculine conditioning and the powerful characteristics or tendencies that influenced his behavior.

Between Him and You:

QUESTION: Why are men often taken in by shallow, manipulative women whom they treat with such respect, whereas they take the caring, nonmanipulative woman for granted?

ANSWER: "Men are easy to manipulate," Sue Ellen, a Texas "blond beauty" told me matter-of-factly. "Most men are starving for a woman to feed their ego, making him feel like he's the best. Successful men are so vulnerable and easy to get to and control that it's hard to understand why some women think men are so difficult. The problem those women have is that they take men too seriously. They're mechanical, love-starved, defensive little boys. If you remember that, act accordingly, and limit your expectations, you can get next to almost any man."

Men have "blind spots" in relating to women and none more clearly demonstrates their personal helplessness and potential self-destructiveness than the compelling power the insincere, manipulative woman has over an otherwise seemingly intelligent man.

The external way most men learn to relate to and experience their personal relationships, where superficial feminine symbols and gestures readily get confused with what the woman is really all about, make men prone to poor choices and self-destructive decisions in relationships.

Few men are able to read behind the smile, seductive and friendly manner, and ego-inflating attention to see the reality of who and what a woman is. Nor can they accurately translate their own feelings or motives. Consequently, in vulnerable moments of loneliness, or the need for validation, the woman who understands what a man "needs"—and gives it to him—can sidetrack him from his course and take over his life.

The ability of the manipulative woman to attract successful, intelligent men is an expression of men's deeper anxieties over personal closeness and the fear of losing control by getting too involved. Because men seek relationships they can "control" and that give them ego gratification and the feeling of real love without genuine personal interaction or demands, they are vulnerable to the woman who is not interested in a relationship either, but wants her needs met, and knows how to give men what they need. She "knows" his vulnerability and limitations and capitalizes on them.

The manipulative woman is an expression of a man's defensively inflated yet very vulnerable ego that, in personal relationships prevents him from distinguishing false responses from those that are sincere.

Thus the manipulative woman is an expression of the tragic flaw that lies at the core of masculinity. The more of "a man" he is, the more his deeper self unconsciously moves toward personal detachment and the less able he is to relate personally.

When men "escape" from the conflicts and boredom of a traditional marriage into the arms of a manipulative woman, they get very excited, thinking they are getting a "fresh start." Instead they become more deeply and firmly entrenched in a personal oblivion and depression.

The unreality and pseudo-excitement created by the popular "centerfold fantasy" also is a symptom of masculine defensiveness. That seeming "excitement" when translated into reality can only produce boredom, volatile miscommunication, mutual exploitation, accusation and, finally, repulsion and despair. Yet men readily succumb to that illusion, even though it defies logic.

The man most vulnerable to attractive bimbos are those who are the most out-of-touch, egotistic, sexually compulsive, immature, self-centered, unable to love and relate personally, aggressive, insecure, and desperate. The bimbo can be the guru that takes him to the bottom of his denied self so he can begin the journey toward nondefensiveness, or she can be one more stopping point on his way to total personal oblivion or the inability to relate personally.

QUESTION: "When we're together, I feel that he wants to be left alone. When I go away, I feel his resentment and the pressure to return. Which one is his true self? Which of the two should I respond to?"

ANSWER: Women who are intensely tuned in to their man become angry and bewildered by the push-pull feelings they get in relating to him.

The conflicting messages men give stem from the defensive aspects of their socialization. On the one hand, men have intense dependency needs that are consciously denied and disguised by an attitude of total self-sufficiency. Once attached to a woman in a relationship, therefore, these deep and intense needs that are extensions of his early fusion with mother, and a lack of bonding with his father, emerge.

Involved with a woman who has a strong need for intimacy, he feels the pressure to be close and personally expressive. So he "closes up" and disconnects. He pushes away to deny his own need, but then his equally great fears of being alone and abandoned return and he pulls her to him. The push-pull is an expression of his inner conflict over his intense unconscious and threatening dependency needs and the need to deny and control them.

I have told many women whose husbands have become emotionally distant and disinterested that the "cure" is to get in touch with their anger at being pushed away, stop pursuing him, and even pull away herself. The moment he senses that, he becomes attentive and she becomes much more appealing. Although this is not a permanent solution, a woman who keeps her distance from a man who resists closeness stands the best chance of getting the intimacy she needs.

There is no simple answer to this dilemma, but the woman who wants to grow and preserve her sense of identity and self-esteem needs to be guided in her responses by the reality of who he is and by the limits of the interaction. This guidance will spare her the pain felt by a woman who "loves too much," where intense efforts at closeness produce the opposite reaction, because she is driven by her needs and not by reality.

It is self-defeating for a woman to accommodate a man's conflicting demands, or to be guided by a desire to be "nice" and loving and to give in to him at the expense of her own identity. Although a man temporarily responds angrily to the woman who *won't* accommodate him, he will be stimulated, threatened, and challenged into becoming his best, potential self. Accommodating his inconsistent demands will only bring out the worst in him.

QUESTION: Why does he talk to me like he would to a child?

ANSWER: The defensive nature of masculinity creates in men a deeply wary and negative experience of the world, which they see as a place where there is never enough power, control, security, or independence. Thus, wealthy, powerful men never seem to get enough wealth or power. Vulnerability, openness, trust, acceptance, submission, and fear are perceived as threatening responses to be avoided.

To the extent that the woman's conditioning produces responses and a worldview that are unlike his; and make her a believer in the power and priorities of love, optimistic about life, with a tendency to focus on the moment rather than the long-range view and to emphasize the personal rather than the external; he believes her to be endangered. Alternately, he may become impatient, protective, critical, patronizing, and paternal.

This dynamic is intensified by the pressures of the male role that cause him to feel responsible for everything and everyone in his personal life. This is reinforced by the tendency of some women in romantic relationships to place responsibilities for decisions and protection on the man.

All of these combined cause him to see her as naive and immature and to react to her in kind.

QUESTION: Why does he forget personal events such as birthdays and anniversaries and even tease me about being too sentimental?

ANSWER: His focus is external and his forgetting reflects his deeper resistance to and disconnection from the personal. In the traditional marriage, the wife even writes the notes and greetings to his parents and family, because he forgets or just doesn't have time to do so. Even the man who remembers sentimental events may do so mechanically, by writing it down and reminding himself so he won't feel guilty or have to face a woman's anger when he forgets.

His primary focus is on the pressures of the "jungle world" of his consciousness. Personal events are distractions from the battle. Getting too involved personally is dangerous—like falling asleep on guard duty.

On the face of it, it seems that little effort is required to remember personal occasions. Yet in light of his conditioning, remembering and doing something about it is a threat to a man's self-protective instincts.

Although this seeming "insensitivity" to personal events may cause pain to his partner, who attaches great significance to them, his forgetful nature or lack of genuine enthusiasm is the price for his "being a man" and is nothing personal.

Although he may have remembered these events more readily during the courtship and romantic period of the relationship, at that time remembering had "a purpose or goal," which was to win and keep her love. Therefore, after marriage his tendency to forget personal events is *not* a sign that he is less involved or "in-love." It is just that his focus has become fully externalized.

QUESTION: How do men really feel about the women they are involved with in relationships?

ANSWER: His responses to a relationship are numerous. Men have an intense need for a "special woman," in order to give meaning to an otherwise disconnected, isolated existence and the pursuit of external goals that can become increasingly meaningless if he is alone.

For many men, his partner is his

personal lifeline. Although the personal stress of the relationship may make it seem that he doesn't care because of his defensive attitude, he does.

In addition, men feel frustrated and angry about their inability to communicate their vision of reality, their values, and their interpretation of life. The hopelessness of the dialogues that go nowhere and often cause a woman to become upset by a man's abrasive style and lead to arguments that never get resolved, generate in him a "giving up" attitude and increasing withdrawal.

Also, there is anxiety concerning a woman's emotional "overreactions" to his missteps. Consequently, men tend to hide feelings from their partner, fearful that she will not understand or that she will overreact. The "big man" afraid of his "little wife" is a common yet accurate stereotype. He is the "bad boy" afraid to be caught with his fantasies, feelings, and motives revealed. He fears that she will never forgive his failings, so he hides them.

Feelings of helpless rage build up in him because of her emotional responses of frustration, anger, and tears brought about by his behaviors. In the face of this he withdraws and feels increasingly "powerless" and controlled.

Boredom may set in because of his need for external stimulation, challenge, and novelty that stand in opposition to the traditional female expectations and direction of a committed love relationship that focuses on just being together.

He is caught in a paradoxical bind. The more she "loves him" and acts accordingly, the more unstimulated he may feel, even though a woman's love is crucial to his well-being.

In the traditional relationship, the notion of love and whether or not it exists, overlooks the complex buildup of many of a man's reactions and feelings because of his nonpersonal upbringing that focuses on achievements, not relationships.

QUESTION: What do men want in a relationship?

ANSWER: What we tell ourselves we want and how we actually respond in a relationship often stand in opposition. What men want is as contradictory as their personalities, where self-sufficiency and dependency create a push-pull, come-here/go-away jumble of responses.

What men want when they are seeking a relationship and what

they want when they are involved in one tends to be different. In the former, he may want attention and intensity; in the latter, he may want just the opposite.

Perhaps a better way to answer this question is to identify the triggers that cause a man to withdraw and to become distant and insensitive. These triggers include:

1. Tears and expressions of pain that he is accused of causing but doesn't understand; and that make him feel unfairly blamed.
2. Criticism of his behavior and the pressure to reassure his partner that love exists without her corresponding awareness of how her responses keep him at arm's length.
3. Assertions that he is selfish and unloving when he believes he is being generous and loving.
4. Criticism of his worldview and response to people as cynical, "sick," or negative without awareness of the pressure he is under to find success in the competitive world.
5. Assertions that he is intentionally making everything

but the relationship his priority.

What brings out the best in him, and triggers his most loving behavior, include:

1. Stimulation and challenges provided by the kind of separate identity and self-esteem of a woman, which makes it "dangerous" for him to withdraw because she will not allow herself to be kept at arm's length.
2. Sufficient inner security on the woman's part so that he does not feel pressured for reassurance. She feels confident in her ability to become fulfilled without his help or presence.
3. Competence and autonomy in his partner that reassure him that he need not feel responsible for her survival or for her happiness, and that she loves him for who he is, not for what he can do or provide.
4. An understanding of his inner conflicts, motives, and struggles that means she will not unfairly interpret or respond to his behavior as being unloving or unfeeling.
5. Overall, a relationship rhythm

that makes it necessary for him to work for involvement rather than take it for granted.

QUESTION: Why does he seem to treat me like an object?

ANSWER: The feeling of being treated like an object is common among women. When men do that, they are unaware of doing so, and thus angry confrontation and accusation only intensify the problem. If sufficiently intimidated by accusations, he may come to hide his true feelings, but no real change has taken place.

As a boy he learns to relate to himself as well as to others by function and goal. For anything or anybody to be allowed into his life, they must serve a purpose. His use of people as objects is unwitting, but a direct expression of being conditioned to have a pragmatic orientation. He applies it to himself as well and thinks of himself in terms of what he does and how well he does it. He is an object in his mind also.

Treating people, including himself, like an object is what being "a real man" is all about. He experiences his physical self as if it were a machine or object composed of disconnected parts. His penis is a piece of plumbing that either "works well" or doesn't. His body is a series of disconnected parts that need to be fixed when he's ill. Emotional problems are the result of irrational thinking, according to him.

He attempts to solve complex personal problems with mechanical solutions and makes matters worse with his need for concrete, logical answers. Even his best friends are really objects—extensions of his golf club, tennis racket, or business ventures.

He gives his children answers to their concerns and lectures about life that suggest they, too, are objects, because his words of advice have little relation to the way they experience themselves and life. He doesn't know them and sees them as extensions of himself, so they feel alienated and irritated by his well-meaning advice and expressions of concern and love.

If and when he seeks help in counseling, he wants answers that exist apart from himself. Life and relationships are like his automobile, which should be "fixed" with external solutions.

In relationships, a man believes he loves a woman as a person and is frustrated and bewildered by accusations that he views her as an object, because the way he "treats" her is the way he has learned, and he is convinced that he treats her much better than anyone else.

QUESTION: Why does he recoil when I tell him that I love him, or when I touch him spontaneously?

ANSWER: It was a shock when men discovered many of the things they did, which they believed were expressions of love, were experienced by women as patronizing acts of chauvinism or as self-serving. Similarly, women do and say things they may believe are loving expressions and that men may even pretend to enjoy. Nonetheless, the tenseness of his body and his self-conscious response when approached spontaneously "for a hug" reveal his underlying discomfort and negative feelings. It is experienced as a jolt, an intrusion, or a demand to respond and get involved.

One man expressed it as, "Her embraces often catch me off guard and while part of me wants to feel it's nice that she loves me and wants to show affection, I feel more irritated than anything else by the suddenness and the expectations and hidden demand that I reciprocate."

A married man echoed this sentiment: "My wife's spontaneous hugs and kisses always feel like a test. Will I return it with enthusiasm? Do I *really* love her? Am I happy that she kissed me?"

QUESTION: Why does he hate it when I cry?

ANSWER: A woman's tears during a stressful discussion feel to a man the way his analytic detachment feels to a woman when something very personal and emotional is being discussed. She experiences it as rejection and a lack of caring even though he would probably see it differently. Similarly, he experiences an emotional outburst as controlling, manipulative, and an indirect attack designed to make him feel guilty, which is why he reacts negatively.

A woman's crying is both an indirect accusation that a man has been hurtful and destructive, and an indirect statement that she sees herself as fragile and abused, which feeds his tendency to feel guilty and responsible for her well-being.

In other words, tears make him feel guilty, manipulated, controlled, and helpless to change things. It is those meanings he conveys to emotional outbursts that create his negative reactions.

In a more profound and critical sense, women's tears under stress symbolize the essential hopelessness of mutually responsible change in the relationship. Men's negative reaction to tears therefore may be a deeper awareness of being in a no-win, escalating situation that spells doom to the future happiness in the relationship.

QUESTION: Why is he afraid to commit?

ANSWER: Men who do not feel threatened are eager to commit. But, like women, men are fearful of being pressured into a relationship where he is an object who must satisfy the needs of his partner.

Women seeking marriage may think of men in terms of their commitment potential. Women upset over a man's reluctance to commit need to ask themselves whether the relationship is a friendship of mutual interest or a power struggle between two people with opposing needs and agendas.

Healthy commitment evolves as a by-product of genuine love and caring. In a true friendship, one does not need to ask for commitment. The relationship will continue to develop because it nourishes both people. When there is pressure to satisfy one person's needs over the other's, the undertow of resentment that builds will undermine the relationship. The woman will suffer from the effects of an absence of genuine desire, whereas the man will feel resentment over having been forced into something he wasn't ready for.

The urgency for commitment is essentially self-serving when it overrides the shared goals of each person, much like sex that is pressured for against the woman's will and desire. Sex or commitment not mutually desired is the use of the other person as an object, and as such contains the seeds of their own destruction.

Men commit readily when they feel safe and nourished. A reluctance to commit is indicative of a relationship with unresolved conflict and issues.

QUESTION: If I'm so important to him, as he says I am, why does he take me for granted and treat me so insensitively?

ANSWER: There are optimal conditions for both sexes under which their capacities for love or sexuality or even rage are maximized. That same insensitive, disinterested man, when his wife pulls away and stops pursuing him, suddenly wakes up and begins to pay attention and show affection.

The sexes often develop polarized distance needs such that, when one is the most urgently involved, albeit for the wrong reasons, the other is shutting down and withdrawing.

In a committed relationship, deeper needs for more intimacy and closeness on the part of a woman arise, and when they do, the "pressure" to respond in a required way cause him to back off. His "harshness" and "insensitivity" can be seen as an unconscious attempt to push away and create a balance that will allow him to remain enthusiastic and stimulated.

In the face of intense intimacy needs, men initially want to respond positively. When they realize they are failing, they begin to drift away. As she becomes more "needy," he becomes more self-protective and a distressing, vicious cycle is set in motion. He can't control this unconscious movement, which expresses itself by his self-absorption, lack of attention, impatience, and irritation.

The cycle of a man's guilt and resentment and a woman's feeling of rejection accelerates as one defensive response triggers another. Each sex needs to be aware of his or her part in the cycle. The undertow, or unconscious distance struggle, is the massive "blind zone" of relationships.

Women can understand this process if they can remember a relationship with a man to whom they felt attracted initially because he was autonomous and strong. Then, when he became insecure and possessive, requiring constant attention, control, and involvement, the love dissolved and caused her to respond unintentionally in cruel and rejecting ways.

QUESTION: Why was he so eager for sex when we first met, and now that we're committed and I really enjoy it and want it, he seems to be indifferent or even tries to avoid it?

ANSWER: Ideas about men's sexuality have developed largely from the old notions of the lusting male and the reluctant, disinterested female. The "horny" male and the "frigid" female are by-products of traditional masculine/feminine polarization and are contingent on men and women relating to each other in traditionally polarized, role-rigid, object-to-object ways.

When that rhythm changes, men's sexuality changes and, when that rhythm reverses, men's sexuality becomes opposite to what it formerly was. In contemporary marriages, the traditional model of a man obsessed with sex because each time he gets it feels like it might be the last, has radically changed.

Today, the woman is no longer the unavailable, resistant object, but someone who actively seeks out an intense closeness and a sexual satisfaction. Under the pressure of her expression of needs, he withdraws and "shuts down." Sexuality is not a challenge, but part of a pressure to be close and involved and to satisfy her. He has lost control of her and the sexuality—a control that had formerly brought his sexual urgency to a fever pitch and kept it there.

Although the ingredients for his sexual urgency sound like a model for male chauvinism, he is as much a "victim" as a "victimizer" in that cycle. To be driven by extreme sexual cravings for a disinterested partner brought out the worst in him in terms of self-destructive and extreme behaviors. Men's true sexuality is far removed from the defensive urgencies of the macho male, where sex became a powerful obsession resulting from the sexual imbalance of the traditional relationship.

To understand the shifting currents of men's sexual desire, look not to the sex itself, but to the balance elements between the sexes. Sex is rarely the real problem, and in healthy male/female relationships it will not have the power to create either the ecstasy or misery it once had.

QUESTION: Why do men have extramarital affairs and should these relationships be taken seriously?

ANSWER: Relationships are constantly in the process of rebalancing themselves and when a relationship is seriously imbalanced or polarized, the search for an escape develops in the partner who is suffering most. An affair acts as a release and an upheaval that can both destroy and restore the relationship if its message is heeded.

When women feel controlled, distanced, and ignored, they are vulnerable to seeking an affair in order to satisfy their frustrated needs for intimacy. Men whose wives have become too dependent and insecure and who no longer provide stimulation that comes from separateness in identity, build up tension and resentment over the engulfment or suffocation. At that point, an affair with a woman who makes no demands and allows the man to maintain his optimal distance is experienced as exciting and irresistible.

To leave a man who cheats or to extract promises of future fidelity, if you stay, misses the point. His affair is a symptom of the imbalance which, if not altered, will cause the cheating to continue.

The cheating itself is rarely an indication of his desire to end a marriage. The other woman is attractive only so long as the urgency of her needs for closeness and commitment have not yet been expressed fully.

Women least likely to be cheated on are those who are the least man-centered, or relationship-focused. When women retain their separate identity, stimulation and balance can be maintained more readily so cheating is not inviting. A relationship-obsessed woman, much like a sex-obsessed man, drives her partner away because the pressure and demands of the underlying insecurity become oppressive.

To leave a relationship for that reason, with only a sense of having been an unfaithful man's victim, overlooks the golden opportunity to learn about oneself and the relationship and truly transform the relationship.

What is needed to keep a man faithful and happy is the wrong question. Sexual excitement cannot be artificially contrived; it exists in proportion to the balance and distance elements of the relationship. When he feels *too much* distance from her ("Maybe she doesn't care or she's interested in someone else"), his sexual interest is very likely to be obsessive. Conversely, when he feels no distance because of her constant demands for reassurance and closeness, his sexual passions may diminish and disappear. At this point, in an attempt to find the distance he needs, another woman will become attractive.

A woman who understands male dynamics will focus on changing the interaction with the man she loves and not choose a punitive solution.

QUESTION: Why do men become so anxious, and even panic-stricken, when they can't perform sexually?

ANSWER: Because of their externalization, men tend to perceive their sexual response in mechanical terms and to lose touch with the messages communicated by the shifts in their potency.

A "balking penis" pushes a man to acknowledge his suppressed feelings and his deeper self, by creating intense anxiety over a response he can't control but needs in order to feel manly. The panic that tends to occur because he has lost control causes him to seek instant cures or solutions. He feels helpless in the face of his impotence because he can't control it by conscious will and it creates intense feelings and concerns that threaten him.

As a therapist for many men who have had sexual dysfunction, I never talk about THE SEX PROBLEM. Instead, we talk about who he is and what his relationship to women is all about. If he can open himself up to that, the so-called sexual problem corrects itself, unless its cause is physiological.

His "dysfunctional" penis is either the beginning of a path back to self-awareness or, if his anxiety level is too high to absorb new awareness, can be the beginning of a downward spiral of anxiety, desperate solutions, self-hate, and depression.

QUESTION: Why does he fall asleep so soon after sex, and does that mean he doesn't love his partner or that he's selfish?

ANSWER: Men who regularly fall asleep after ejaculation are making a statement that reflects their mechanical way of relating, and the minimal personal nature of the relationship.

If ejaculation means he got what he needed—specifically sexual release—and he needs to avoid the process of being close, then he is likely to fall asleep. His response is beyond his awareness, intention, or control. Negative confrontations, hurt feelings, and accusations of selfish disinterest only promote guilt and further alienation.

The relationship needs work for both partners, but feeling used or rejected is counterproductive because he does not intend to be insensitive or hurtful. However, if the message is that he is too self-absorbed to fulfill his partner's needs, she needs to recognize the state of the relationship and insist on therapeutic efforts to change it, or consider leaving.

QUESTION: Why doesn't he like to go on vacations even though he works so hard?

ANSWER: Vacations have the same "feel" for men as other activities such as shopping do. Vacations are a distraction from the "serious" pursuits of life that constantly preoccupy him. Therefore, if he had his way, according to how he honestly felt, he might *never* go on a vacation.

The problems and conflicts in a relationship are harder to disguise on vacations. At home, constant daily responsibilities allow him to avoid these problems. In addition, the more dangerous life feels to him, the more being away from the battle creates anxiety. Thus the longer vacations continue, the more he will feel irritable and threatened, looking for reasons to "escape" back into work.

Vacations highlight the depth and intensity of the male/female differences in a relationship. Couples in a balanced relationship have fun. Extremely polarized couples experience extreme agony. "Vacations are hell" is how one traditional male described it. Another remarked, "Vacations are exhausting. It's great to get back to work—and relax."

QUESTION: Why are men so insensitive in their personal relationships?

ANSWER: It is one of the paradoxes of a

man's conditioning that the same aspects of his manliness that initially make him so attractive, come to be experienced as insensitivities when he is in an ongoing relationship. Once committed, Prince Charming seems to transform into Mr. Rat in his partner's eyes. That which was initially positive transforms into a negative.

His logical, cool, and controlled manner are experienced as a lack of feeling, coldness, and fear of intimacy. His decisive, take-charge manner emerges as an oppressive need to control his partner and a "disinterest" in what she wants. His independent, self-sufficient style becomes a distant, withdrawn manner which makes his partner feel rejected and unneeded. His ambitious goal direction and competitiveness make him seem selfish, aggressive, and unloving as the relationship evolves.

Men in relationships are bewildered by the shift away from romantic feelings during courtship toward critical, negative interpretations of him later on, and how his partner seems to become so easily provoked and angry.

"I haven't changed, yet somehow everything she loved about

me initially seems to enrage her now. I'm the same, but her so-called love for me certainly isn't," is how one man summed it up.

Between Him and Others:

QUESTION: Why doesn't he like his father?

ANSWER: "I don't call my dad when something good happens to me," stated a young man of twenty-nine. "I call Mom. If I tell my dad, I don't sense any real joy or excitement. Sometimes he'll even make a cynical comment like, 'You're finally getting somewhere,' or he'll say, 'That's great son!' and change the subject."

Violent male criminals often have tattoos with a heart and arrow that says MOM. Tearfully, they apologize for the heartache they've caused her. Mention Dad, and they express hatred and even a wish to kill him "if I ever see him again." From their macho perspective, Mom was a saint and Dad a cold bastard.

Little boys get the brunt of their father's negative and defensive perceptions of the world. In preparing their sons for a world they perceive negatively, they alienate them and drive them away and closer still to their mothers. This creates in the boy an explosive macho defensiveness because of his intense need to prove his masculinity and deny the deep identification and powerful attachment to his mother. The young boy hasn't identified himself with the dad he fears and hates, sees as cold and critical, and yet has to please and emulate out of fear. Emotional impenetrability and conditional love based on performance are what Dad is all about to most young boys.

Fathers fail to know who their sons are in their urgency to transform them into high-performance, fearless machines. When a father thinks he's talking to his son, often he's deluded. He is not being heard because of the inner wall his son is building up to avoid his critical manner.

The more pressuring a father is, the more the young boy will move toward his mother emotionally. She, in turn, may try to meet some of her own needs for closeness and affection through her relationship with her son, an intimacy she isn't getting from Dad either.

The more traditional Dad is, the more the young boy's attitude toward life is like his mother's because his emotional attachment and therefore identification are with her. Because she feels controlled, frustrated, hurt, and angry at Father (even though she might deny it), her son comes to empathize with her, and unconsciously shares her rage and frustration in her relationship with Dad.

Because of his intense bonding with his mother and alienation from his father, he cannot understand or empathize with him. Thus he blames his father for the problems in the family also. As an adult he may cover it up, but his extreme disconnection toward his father reveals his absence of loving emotion.

A father's "error of projection" is such that the harder he pushes his son to be a man, the less of a "real man" the boy is actually going to become. In extremely polarized homes, what is produced is a violent macho son, uncontrollable in his explosive need to prove his manliness because he identifies with his mother.

QUESTION: Why doesn't he have any close friends?

ANSWER: The quality of men's personal interaction with each other is fragile despite a surface veneer of camaraderie and buddyship. Trust among men is easily shattered; conversations readily run dry as each tends to communicate externally (two machines talking) without personal sharing. The impersonal nature of their interactions places serious limits on the pleasure and fulfillment of being together.

Most men have "activity friends"—men who are extensions of their interests in sports such as tennis, golf, football, or in other external interests. When the activity is absent, the pleasure in and reasons for continuing the relationship usually dissolve. Devoid of a personal foundation, the absence of a shared activity is the death knell of the relationship. With nothing external to channel them, the interaction ceases.

As boys, males learn to interact with others for a purpose. Otherwise, they retreat into themselves and into the pursuit of skills development and achievement. As boys they are taught that they need to be doing something or interacting for a reason. An additional disconnecting element is the endless pressure to prove himself as a performer, which always focuses him on future events in order to maintain and build his self-esteem and image.

As an adult, marriage tends to provide a reason to close off any remaining friendship bonds. He may feel guilty leaving his wife to go off with a buddy to have fun when she tells him that he rarely spends any leisure time with her.

As men get older, they become more withdrawn from personal relationships. The fantasy of male bonding and camaraderie has its basis in truth only in situations where there is a shared goal or target (enemy). When those "reasons" dissolve, so does the so-called men's club.

QUESTION: Why do men seem so negative and cynical about people and life once you get to know their real feelings?

ANSWER: The cynical worldview, which tends to intensify as men get older, regardless of whether a facade of conviviality and "nice guy" behavior exists, can best be understood by recognizing the psychological components that make up his conditioning as a man.

His defensive autonomy generates an accompanying feeling in him that he is alone and no one really cares, knows him, or can be depended on if he becomes sick or vulnerable.

The defensive aggression that makes him ambitious and competitive is unconsciously projected, and so he sees the world as a jungle and most people as a threat if he makes himself vulnerable.

His need to achieve and validate himself by being productive causes others to relate to him on the basis of what he can do and provide. He becomes cynical about "love" when he sees them relate to him positively when they want something, but ignore him when they don't. When he no longer provides, he believes he will be rejected.

His need to control and his fear of submission and weakness alienates others and he eventually accepts this loveless state as the price of security.

The same components that make him attractive as a man, create this veil of negativity. The realities he creates around himself, in the outside as well as his personal world, continually confirm his most negative attitudes about life. He can't understand how his defensiveness has created these attitudes, because they are by-products of his process. Therefore he believes his view of the world is objective and accurate.

QUESTION: Why is he still so insecure, even though he's successful?

ANSWER: Just as many women feel that they are never quite thin enough or beautiful enough, many men never feel secure, powerful, or rich enough even though it doesn't make rational sense to an outside observer.

The drive to be "successful" comes from the insatiable defensive motivations of his masculine being, much like his need to prove his masculinity. The insecurities that create his compulsions also create the process of an increasing isolation and disconnection. This makes him feel more vulnerable as he gets older, and so he needs "more" to feel secure and to protect himself. His world is one in which a lifetime of winning in his mind, can be undermined by a moment of inattention or letting down his guard.

Success actually becomes easier to achieve as personal disconnection and resistance to closeness increases. Working, acquiring *MORE*, becomes the tranquilizer that relaxes him and makes him feel safe. As his world gets "colder" he tries to warm it up with a more intense pursuit of *more*, that he believes will bring love, respect, and appreciation but bring about the opposite—the resentments, jealousies, and hostilities of those around him.

Each higher level of success raises his standard for failure; a standard that is his own. The "illogic" of men's quests that intensifies his insecurity is that the process of pursuing his goals alienates the very people he tells himself he is doing it all for. As he becomes more successful, therefore, personal relationships become more fragile and loss of power stands as an ever greater threat of exposing just how alone and alienated he really is. With more success he believes he will have more control and will eventually be able to change the pattern. It doesn't happen, however, and the feelings engendered cause him to strive for more self-protection. It is a vicious cycle.

QUESTION: Why is he so moody: first high and happy and then suddenly in a bad mood, and for no apparent reason?

ANSWER: Although the up-and-down cycle of men's moods sounds like a definition of manic-depression, the "moodiness" of a man exists in proportion to his externalization (how dependent on outside events he is), which makes his self-esteem and sense of security vulnerable to and dependent on the slightest alterations in his performance and external fortunes.

His is a "self" that readily "bounces off walls." Observe, for example, the intensely competitive tennis player and his euphoria after making a good shot, followed soon by disgust, rage, and self-condemnation after a few missed or poor shots. Or, observe the man who experiences impotency after years of performing adequately. His self-esteem plummets. "I'm not the man I was," he concludes. His response can be so despairing and self-loathing that one might think he had never had successful sex. His mood swings are a direct expression of that expanding/contracting sense of himself.

Because his ego is always on the line, he readily gives up endeavors, interests, and pursuits he can no longer perform adequately. He can't tolerate doing something badly, even if it's just for pleasure.

For these reasons, an inner cycle that goes from "I'm the greatest!" to a despairing, "I'm nobody," can occur quickly for seemingly insignificant reasons. Performance is what defines him as "a man," and the lack of performance robs him of that feeling.

As he gets older, his battles become more difficult because he has become isolated and alienated and his capacities are diminishing. As a result the changes in mood may become even more extreme and sudden. The so-called wisdom of old age in men is a fantasy. The reality is the opposite: with age his increasing defensiveness makes him more rigid and less able to control his moods.

QUESTION: If men want to be close to their families, why don't they make that a priority?

ANSWER: Most men are convinced that they are making their families their priority. They have learned to love by doing, earning, protecting, advising, making decisions, and such—not by personal relating. When they do these things, they expect to be loved and appreciated in return. The bond is tenuous, however, because in the process of fulfilling his role, disconnection rather than closeness is operating. So, the wife and children he is "doing it all for" become strangers who may resent him for not having been there, for giving unwanted advice, and for being critical, preoccupied, negative, and aloof. What he has done seems to count for almost nothing because no intimate attachment has occurred.

Successful men, because their success is in proportion to their externalization and disconnection, suffer the most from the paradox of having "given the most" and being "loved the least," or resented, even hated for being controlling, insensitive, critical, cold, and so on. This only serves to confirm to such men what an unloving place the world is—a place where only external power is respected.

The essential illogic of men's logic, their obvious blind spot, is apparent as they continue to do those things that clearly don't work, in the hopes of somehow making them work. He is trapped and doesn't know how to get out, which is one reason men suddenly self-destruct, leave home, or become ill. It is a response to the futility of the process they are in.

QUESTION: Why does he dislike shopping?

ANSWER: Just as men and women love differently, they shop differently. Women shop for recreation and pleasure, whereas most men shop with a definite goal or purpose in mind. Men's perception of women's shopping is probably comparable to women's perception of men's relationship to work. "Oh, no! Not again!! What for?"

His conditioning creates in him a denial of personal needs. Shopping is an acknowledgment of needs. Although the traditional man can buy for others, he may have difficulty spending money on himself unless he can justify it for functional reasons. The same pair of shoes might be worn until they fall apart, unless his work demands otherwise.

Shopping may trigger his negative views of the world also. "They only try and sell you junk that you don't need, so that they can get your money." Because most women don't experience the world cynically, such preoccupations rarely occur and they are able to enjoy buying beautiful new things.

5

Shared Struggles/ Polarized Realities

Timothy, a thirty-nine-year-old teacher, described the process of breaking through damaging patterns that had destroyed his first two marriages—both of which began on high romantic notes and ended with bitterness and accusation.

Determined not to repeat these patterns, he began psychotherapy to learn about what he was doing to hurt and anger women, and how he could relate to a woman as a person rather than as a prize. He had always been drawn to "flashy, sexy, head-turning women."

Soon after beginning counseling, he dated a woman and for the first time remained in the relationship even though there was no initial romantic rush. "She was easy to be with, someone who seemed to know how to be a friend and a good playmate. We laughed a lot on dates. When we spent weekends together, I didn't get bored; and I didn't feel I had to entertain her or do the usual—going to restaurants and movies. We didn't have to busy ourselves with entertainment to enjoy each other, so I knew that this might be special and new for me."

Nevertheless, there was still a struggle to prevent the relationship from taking a traditional path. "I had become much less interested in being in control and, in fact, had gotten to the point where I enjoyed being the passive receiver at least as much as the initiator. Nevertheless, even though Allison was a strong person, I could feel the tension when I waited for her to make the decisions, and let her lead the way. Other times she would take full responsibility and make the decisions and I could feel myself resisting and faking feeling good by acting pleased and cooperative even though I really felt pushed and irritated.

"I'd want her to pay her own way, and then I'd feel guilty when she did. Or I could see her discomfort when she paid more than once in a day, like for the theater and an after-theater drink, even though she would deny that.

"I'd want her to be sexually assertive yet I'd find myself wishing we'd have sex only when I initiated it, because when she'd initiate, I'd find myself less excited, even though I pretended to be pleased because I didn't want to be the selfish male. There were many other instances where just really being friends and not playing the traditional man/woman games that I'd played at and gotten in trouble with in past relationships seemed confusing and very hard. I'd catch myself longing for the old ways and would have to remind myself how boring and destructive they were. I can understand why the old way is hard to give up, though. It's the line of least resistance, and it's nice to believe you might make it work 'this time,' just to get out of doing the hard work of dealing with the tensions and conflicts as they come up."

Shared Struggles

Whatever women struggle with, men struggle with the opposite. Although one partner's behavior may have a better surface appearance in a given situation, the sexes trigger each other in a reciprocal dance of polarized opposites. The result is painful, problematic, and hurtful to both, even though one partner might be labeled the good guy and the other as the spoiler or the destructive one.

The sense of powerlessness and feelings of being exploited and patronized that women experience in the competitive workplace are matched by the powerlessness, vulnerability, and fragile-volatile quality men experience in their personal lives. It is not unusual to find adult men who have alienated all those who were close to them, including their children, and they can't comprehend why. Commonly, men misread and mismanage the personal relationship they depend on most. A man's most sincere efforts at fulfilling his role obligations may only result in his being disliked or ignored. Most men seem unable to make any personal connection they can fully trust and share their feelings with, particularly when they need help. Thus, instead of reaching out, they withdraw even more just when they need closeness the most.

These are not justifications or apologies for men's limited and inadequate relationship behaviors. Rather, they are examples of a shared struggle—men as counterpart victims of their gender conditioning, which has made them as powerless in personal relationships as they are in control in the impersonal work arena.

The reciprocity of gender problems exists in many areas. Although women are frustrated and alienated by men's fear of closeness and lack of warmth, men speak with frustration and react negatively to what they experience as women's unceasing need for reassurance and warmth. They feel the hopelessness and irrationality of trying to satisfy these needs and to prove that their love is genuine.

Similarly, while women fear men's anger and violence, men feel alienated by women's tears, resistance to negotiating, and the accusations that make him feel that he is the sole cause of the problems.

Women are repelled by men's impersonal sexual obsession, whereas men feel manipulated by women's "use" of their sexuality for control, or as a reward for men's love and involvement.

Women are oppressed by men's defensive egos and their need to control. Men despair over women's resistance to making decisions, clearly stating preferences, and reluctance to take control so that he does not need to feel responsible for his partner's well-being and happiness.

Women feel rejected and alienated by men's preoccupation with work, and numerous other ways of withdrawing from intimacy. Men are exasperated by women's unrealistic attitude toward money, obsession with diets and shopping, and their relentless preoccupation with the relationship.

Each sex struggles to accept and respond positively to the alienating behaviors of the other. Similarly, each responds initially in a favorable way to the feminine or masculine qualities of the other, but eventually feels oppressed and rejected by these very same qualities, which were so attractive at first, but turn out to be annoying and rigid.

For every complaint of one sex there seems to be an equivalent counterpart complaint. Therefore, when relationships turn sour, that quality that was initially so attractive in one partner becomes irritating and offensive. Each accuses the other of deliberately undermining the relationship, refusing to change in order to make things better, and of being "uncaring," "deliberately hurtful," or "crazy."

Only cynics would maintain that men and women enter relationships with a desire to be abusive or hurtful. Yet that is how each partner comes to view the other. The fact that many relationships often end in an unpleasant, antagonistic atmosphere tells us that something in them is seriously out of control, and that the best intentioned behaviors of each partner have backfired. Both are "victims" of an unconscious cycle; yet couples rarely see themselves as equal participants in creating the good as well as the bad, so they go from partner to partner, thinking that things will get better.

To the degree that either sex perceives itself as right or less responsible for the relationship's destruction, relationships will continue their negative, alienating spiral. To effect authentic change, each sex must focus on its own defensive processes, imbalance, projections, distortions, and collusion with the games the sexes play.

In tandem, in the traditional relationship process a man hurts her with his coldness and disconnection; she hurts him by her "hot" emotionalizing and pressuring for an intimacy he is unable to give her. He hurts her with his need for control and his lack of tolerance for being "wrong" or submissive, whereas she hurts him with false accommodation and the loss of her identity to the "we" of the relationship, and a resistance to making decisions, taking initiative, stating preferences, and negotiating for and holding fast to what she feels is important.

A man hurts a woman with his negativity, cynicism, and distrust of people and emotions, whereas she alienates and irritates him with relentless "positive thinking," "naive" optimism about people and problems, "niceness," gullibility concerning authority figures and "gurus," all of which intensify his sense of vulnerability and responsibility for both. He scares her with his eruptions of anger and aggressiveness, whereas she alienates him with her excessive fears, tears, and indications of helplessness, anxiety, and powerlessness.

Men alienate women with their sexual fixations on women as objects for sexual pleasure, whereas women alienate men with their use of sex for reward and control.

A woman feels rejected by a man's resistance to making a total relationship commitment or becoming intimate, whereas a woman distorts the relationship process by pressuring for an intensity of involvement and commitment that is premature, particularly when she threatens to leave him for not giving her what she wants.

He irritates her with his "insatiable" need for material security (money) and power, where there never seems to be enough to ensure the future, whereas she exasperates him with her lack of planning and preparing for the future and her Pollyannaish belief that "everything will be all right," and that "things will work out for the best," which he translates as making him responsible for everything, or no planning will occur.

He wounds her with harsh criticism of her competence, whereas she sets the stage for disappointment by perceiving him as far stronger and more capable of dealing with life than he actually is, and adoring him at first as different from other men, but then resenting him for not turning out as she had imagined him.

A man fuels a woman's insecurity with his silences, lack of emotion, and withdrawal when there is a problem, whereas a woman provokes a man by constantly pressuring him for an openness, closeness, and involvement just at those times he is least able to open up.

A man alienates a woman with his analytic, logical, and mechanical approach to their personal problems, whereas a woman frustrates a man by making "irrational" assertions, unsubstantiated accusations, and pressuring with demands that seem to him unfounded, unreasonable, and provocative.

These together create a relationship cycle where:

1. Women are hurt because they seem to love too much, and men are hurt because they seem to be unable to love.
2. Women are plagued by an excess of external fears and denial of their power; and men destroy themselves by a denial of fears and

vulnerability and an exaggerated sense of their invincibility, and their need to be in control.

3. Women become frustrated and hurt by intense needs and longings for intimacy, which never get satisfied, and men come to feel rejected, lonely, and cynical about love because of an inability to acknowledge or communicate their personal needs.
4. Women are threatened by an identity that is lost and a low level of self-esteem as they become mired in a relationship; and men risk making serious misjudgments because of an inflated ego that demands feeding and validation, and they alienate others with their need to dominate and control.
5. Men are deluded in their belief that logic, truth, and external solutions will transform their personal lives, and women are deluded in their belief that love and faith will provide the answers to their problems.
6. Men are rendered hollow and dehumanized by their approach to reality and meaning through cold objectivity and analysis, whereas women are rendered helpless and vulnerable to manipulation and control by their attraction to and often unquestioning belief in the romantic, psychic, and spiritual.
7. Men enter into the paranoid consciousness of insatiable pursuits of power and material wealth and are trapped by them, whereas women develop an undue sense of helplessness and are victimized by a resistance and inability to access their own aggression

and power; they often tend to blame men for the problems of the world.

8. Men's life purposes are belied by an absence of intimate and caring bonds to the children, family, and friends they provide for, whereas women's lives are limited by an overly intense and close bond with their children—whom they may smother and weaken—and a lack of sufficient involvement with the outside world.

Equal Players

Once having read men's accounts of their relationships in several male periodicals, Beth, a thirty-seven-year-old married mother of two boys, changed her interpretations of and attitudes toward men.

"The evidence is too overwhelming," she said, "to deny that men are victims of their conditioning every bit as much as women are. I read of the men who lose custody of their children and soon find that the children they loved and worked for don't want to see them anymore because they have a new daddy. I think of the divorced men I know who are living lonely lives in small apartments with nobody ever calling to find out if they're alive."

Beth continued, "I see the men who give their lives to the corporation and then suddenly lose their jobs because the company's been bought out and these men don't know what to do with themselves and no one cares when they're let go at some unemployable age.

"All those boys having to be macho and destroying their lives in gangs because they don't know any other way to relate and get approval, and they feel that they *have* to prove their manliness continually. As a woman, I feel a lot of pain and disappointment in my personal life, and in the competitive marketplace. Men obviously go through an awful lot too. They just seem to be less able to articulate it, so it's harder to see."

Although the deterioration process of a relationship usually places the guilt more heavily on one than the other, on a deeper level both are equal players in the downfall—even though one may appear to be more involved and loving and the other more hurtful; or one is passive and the other active in bringing about the destruction. Both have the potential to break the destructive cycle by changing their rooted response, but neither seems to learn from past conflicts and arguments, and each partner continues to repeat the same alienating behaviors.

Understand Him and You'll Understand Yourself

Unwitting defensiveness that comes from polarized conditioning creates opposing "hot spots" or triggers. The tendency toward low self-esteem, created by feminine conditioning, is fueled by the inflated sense of self and power that blocks a man's capacity to listen and relate to others. This causes a woman to feel that a man is discounting her and being overly critical, and prevents a man from recognizing his alienating impact.

A man's denial and resistance to being dependent and vulnerable cause him to overreact defensively when he experiences pressure to be close, which clashes with the woman's need for intimacy and reassurance. It causes her to react to what she perceives as rejection and a lack of caring. One triggers the other. Unwittingly, she pushes him further away, which in turn causes her to feel more insecure, which in turn alienates him.

A woman's discomfort with aggressive behavior creates a desire for everything to be "nice," a denial of her anger, and a tendency to feel powerless and fearful, and resistant to confrontation and conflict. It has a counterpart in the man's defensive tendency to be overly aggressive and to deny fear, which makes him self-destructive. His aggressiveness causes her to be unduly fearful of him and for him to feel self-loathing and guilt for being so destructive when he is unable to control his anger and to acknowledge vulnerability.

A man's fear of seeming submissive creates a defensive "nobody-tells-me-what-to-do" attitude and a tendency to impose his will. This is equivalent to a woman's tendency to resist taking control, only to feel she is powerless and being controlled, and to blame the man for deliberately trying to destroy her identity. He has a "hot spot" about losing control, whereas her "hot spot" involves feeling controlled and violated because she can't take control.

A man's compulsion to always be doing something and to feel useless and anxious when he can't, has a counterpart in a woman's tendency to put a priority on being together as *the* way to express love, and her passive attitude toward initiating activities.

She tends, therefore, to become irritated when she feels his pressure to be active and his insinuations that she is being "lazy" or "useless" because she is not sufficiently goal-driven, like him. In contrast, he feels pressured and alienated by her desire to "just be together." A typical defensive perception was articulated by one man: "She walks a mile every day for exercise, but then she sits and watches soap operas and eats chocolates for hours"; and the counterpart female observation that, "Sure, he'll be with me for a few minutes, but then he has to go out and jog for five miles and get away, or he's half watching TV news while we're in the middle of a conversation."

His tendency to conceal his emotions causes him to be perceived as cold and uncaring, and causes him to overreact defensively to her expressed feelings and thus to see her as "irrational."

In each of these polarizations and in countless variations on the theme of polarized cycles, the defensive extreme of one sex triggers a counterpart extreme reaction in the other, until finally a total polarization has been created and romance is replaced by "hot spots" and mutual triggers that produce constant anger, frustration, and hopelessness about ever improving the relationship.

Without a separate awareness in each stage of this reciprocal defensive cycle, and of how each partner has to change in order to avoid it, the relationship ends in turmoil, where just being together becomes painful, injurious, and dangerous to each partner's psychological well-being.

The Problem of Projection: Believing the Other Person Can Be Like You and Could Change "If They Only Really Wanted To"

Projection is the unconscious, defensive process that makes each partner feel that the other one could be different if they really wanted to, and that they continue to behave as they do because they just don't care. This intensifies the alienation, because each is convinced that the other is being "deliberately" hurtful. Consequently, neither partner learns from the angry encounters, which thus are unproductive and hurtful and have a "grinding down" effect on the relationship.

Neither seems to recognize how their response triggers the reaction that infuriates them. The more he is detached and coldly logical in an attempt to be "reasonable," the more she will become emotional because of feelings of frustration and rejection. The more she responds emotionally, the colder and more detached he becomes, and so it goes.

Neither sees that the other cannot change in the relationship alone, and that without a mutual process of working to reduce the polarization, no permanent or real change can take place. To make matters worse, neither sees how he or she is demanding changes that the other is unable to make in a vacuum, because the response is a part of a mutually triggered cycle.

The unquestioned clichés involving love and relationships hasten the breakdown. Commonly believed notions such as, "underneath it all, men and women are the same," and that "everybody needs love," suggest that if men and women are really sincere, problems could be solved by being caring and loving. They can't. The polarization process is deeply rooted and requires significant self-awareness and growth and a willingness to work hard to change, for improvement to occur.

In romantic relationships, men and women tend to be opposites and counterparts, which is initially compelling but ultimately devastating. Although both partners may need love, their definition of love turns out to be quite different. Sitting down and discussing the problem is rarely enough.

The cliché that "without love there is nothing" suggests that men and women are capable of loving and mutual sharing, which, in traditional relationships, is untrue. Only nonpolarized partners who can relate as good friends can love without generating frustration, defensiveness, and miscommunication.

The solution to breaking through the polarized cycle requires that both partners understand their equal part in the shared struggle—the way each impacts the other and triggers the negative response. Focusing on the other person's irritating response without an equal recognition on one's own accelerates the relationship's destruction.

Laurie, a nurse in her mid-thirties, had a long history of unhappy relationships in which she allowed herself to be "taken from" by a series of men who seemed totally self-centered and exploitative. After a year of therapy, she met a man who seemed to be "different." He was more caring and willing to share than any she'd ever been involved with. He went out of his way to be with her, even if only for a few hours, whereas the men in her past had always expected her to meet them—at their convenience. He was willing to spend money on her, whereas the men in her past never seemed to have any money.

After three months of intense involvement, however, he seemed to change. She discovered that he'd had a couple of "meaningless" sexual experiences with women he'd met at business conferences. He went away on two weekend trips without inviting her. She thought, "Oh, no, I've drawn the same kind of man *again!* I was just kidding myself."

In fact, she hadn't. Rather, her low self-esteem and desperate attempt to make the relationship work at all costs had polarized her new boyfriend and caused him unconsciously to back off and escape from an interaction that had become intimate and intertwined much too quickly, and without a proper foundation.

What changed this time, and set the relationship back on track, was Laurie's ability to recognize that she hadn't attracted the same kind of man again. Rather, she had helped to generate the same kind of defensive withdrawal as she had in the past by relating in an urgent, selfless, and overly intense way.

When Laurie realized this, and instead of blaming her partner began to reestablish her boundaries and stopped "giving too much" to a man who didn't deserve such selflessness, the excitement returned; the damage was undone because the process was changing without either partner being blamed for anything.

The Nonpolarized Healthy Relationship

When a relationship is healthy, meaning that it is not polarized such that the two people can see the other for who and what they are because there is no underlying defensiveness, it has a strong immune system. Like a healthy body, it can absorb blows and traumas and bounce back quickly, without lasting effects or permanent damage resulting from a conflict or problem.

When a relationship is debilitated by polarization, however, and the communication is characterized by blame, guilt, overreactions, and defensive self-justification, it is damaged, and even relatively minor "injury," such as a poorly chosen word or "insensitive" action, can trigger a destructive, negative cycle, which signals the final collapse of the relationships.

The Drugs of Gender: The Counterpart Tranquilizers of Polarized Tensions

When gender needs are defensive (i.e., a man's need for distance, a woman's need "to be close."), tensions build up when playing out or expressing polarized needs is blocked. Men and women both harbor underlying painful feelings and frustrations that cause them to turn to substitute outlets for relief. A man's need to get distance ("disconnect") might be expressed by staying glued to TV sports, endlessly working, or excessive drinking. A woman's frustrated craving for intimacy and love might be ameliorated by shopping for a new dress or a binge on sweets—which serve as consolation and forms of "self-loving."

Each partner tends to criticize the other for these tension-relieving behaviors, seeing them as willful acts rather than as unconscious tranquilizers. The more polarized a person and his or her relationship is, the more widespread and intense will be the use of these "gender tranquilizers."

Here are some common accusatory reactions of partners to each other's alienating or polarizing tension-relieving behaviors.

SHE: You're *always* working.
HE: You're *always* shopping.
SHE: You're *always* watching sports on TV.
HE: You're *always* watching soap operas and those insipid talk shows.
SHE: You're *always* worrying about money.

HE: You're *always* worrying about your weight.

SHE: You're *always* looking for reassurance that there's enough security.

HE: You're *always* looking for reassurance that I love you and that you won't be left.

SHE: You're *always* so cynical.

HE: Everything is *always* so "nice" and "wonderful" in your eyes.

SHE: You're *always* saying you have to stop drinking.

HE: You're *always* saying you have to stop eating.

SHE: You *always* want to be alone.

HE: You *always* want to be together.

SHE: You're *always* reading newspapers and military novels.

HE: You're *always* reading fashion magazines and romance novels.

SHE: You're *always* so quiet. You never want to talk.

HE: You're *always* talking! You won't let me just think.

Addictive behaviors that result from gender tension produce rigid, defensive behavior patterns that grow more extreme and mutually defensive with time. These patterns become so entrenched and are so common in "normal" society they are not taken seriously or studied or understood as being serious, widespread conditions that most of us suffer from in one form or another. Nor are they recognized for what they are: symptoms of the very same underlying process that causes men and women initially to find each other so attractive.

Only when they are so obviously extreme that they threaten the lives and well-being of one or both partners are they finally acknowledged as serious addictions. Even then the causes are sought in each person's early background rather than in the gender conditioning that effects us all and makes us "victims" in one way or another, regardless of our early background.

Although the addictions feel acceptable to the "addicted person," they are irritating and alienating to the partner and generate endless futile discussions with the intent to change the other person by trying to convince them about the destructiveness of their behavior.

Each of the partners finds themselves making the same speeches repeatedly. She tells him, "What's the point of always working and earning more money if our relationship is going to pot," *or* "You don't seem to trust or like anybody. You have a major problem and you'd better work on it."

His speeches to his partner are equally as predictable and ineffective. "God, you're on another diet. Why don't you just develop some sensible habits?" *or*, "Just because I'm not always hugging you or saying 'I love you,' doesn't mean I don't care. How often do I have to prove that to you?"

But because they are addictions, resolutions to change don't last and the behaviors tend to become more frequent, rigid, and extreme with time.

Men rationalize their addictions. Workaholism and "exercise-aholism" are rationalized as "positive addictions," because they temporarily produce positive results even as they ultimately disconnect and alienate men in their personal relationships. Women rationalize their addictions to "love," "intimacy," food, clothes, obsessive grooming, and such, as being what they need in order to feel good. Each partner can see through the rationalizations and self-delusions of the other, but not their own.

The addictive behaviors are the tension relievers we come to crave. They are tranquilizing agents for gender tensions and frustrations. When we can't indulge them, we become irritated, and unhappy, even desperate. The man who yells at his wife and children for interrupting him as he watches still another ball game, or spends his leisure time working out or reading money reports, resenting any intrusion from family or friends, can't see the damaging process and destructiveness of these behaviors. Similarly, the woman who craves constant hugs and reassurances of love, or who spends hours obsessing about her appearance, doesn't see the self-defeating nature of her defensive process. What is supposed to reassure her of love and her beauty actually does the opposite.

The addiction is seen when finally he becomes totally focused on his work and feels good only when he's engaged in some such "productive," goal-directed activity; and she becomes addicted to her pursuits to the exclusion of everything else. When their relationship has been destroyed, each feels embittered and betrayed, and unable to understand their part in the alienating process. Instead, they come to view their partner as an enemy, who was deliberately hurtful and lacking in compassion and understanding.

For the man who is not addicted to eating and dieting, or to shopping, astrology, or daytime TV, these preoccupations seem irrational but easy to control. The woman who is not addicted to TV sports, exercise, work, money, or "doing something" can't understand these compulsions in a man and sees him as doing them deliberately and for selfish reasons. For the partner who does not develop the underlying tension that demands relief, the habits that develop to ease them seem self-centered and deliberate.

Another Shared Struggle: We Both Feel Criticized and Attacked

The polarization process causes both sexes to feel misunderstood and insensitively treated. It produces a cycle of blaming and self-justification:

"She doesn't understand me."
"He's always putting me down."
"I'm never good enough for her."
"He can't give me what I need."
"She tells me I don't really love her and that I'm self-centered and only love myself."
"He doesn't appreciate all of the love and attention I give him. There's no point in continuing."
"She thinks my success is just a successful manipulation of others."
"He doesn't know how to relate."
"She minimizes the things I give her—and blows out of proportion what I'm not so good at."

"He doesn't really listen to anything I say."
"She tells me I'm totally insensitive. I don't know what that means."
"He says it should be enough that he's a good provider and doesn't cheat on me. It's not."
"It's never enough for her. There's always something more that she needs.

Women feel rejected when men do not welcome the intensity of their emotional involvement. He says, "All she thinks about is the relationship and whether it's any good." Men are angered when women do not value their efforts at providing material necessities and comforts. She says, "I'd rather have less materially and more closeness." He can't hear that, and continues on, feeling misunderstood, thereby reinforcing her belief that he really doesn't care.

Men are bewildered when women they really care for tell them that they feel unfairly criticized, attacked, discounted, taken for granted, and not really loved. He seems unable to understand how his unconscious tendency to lecture and his attempts to be "helpful" by telling her how to do something are seen as criticism. It conveys the message that he really doesn't know what her priorities are and that he doesn't understand her. Unknowingly, he comes across as trying to make her over as something she is not, when he believes that he is only trying to be loving and helpful.

Women feel frustrated, rejected, and angry when the priority they place on love, intimacy, and the quality of the relationship is perceived as neurotic and pressuring.

A sense of futility occurs in men when their

attempts to be giving and loving are perceived as criticisms, whereas women begin to feel hopeless when their attempts to discuss the relationship and personal feelings in order to create more closeness are minimized and ignored.

Both develop a sense of futility about having what each believes to be their message of love, goodwill, and caring misconstrued. Because of the polarized realities, the message of each is perceived as the reverse of what was intended by the giver. The breakdown in communication goes both ways, as the polarized experiences of reality cause communication to be distorted.

- He thinks he's being responsible when he makes work a priority, whereas she sees it as an escape from the relationship.
- She thinks that she's being loving and giving when she makes the relationship her priority, whereas he sees it as pressuring and an attempt to avoid the other, more important responsibilities.
- He doesn't want to be told that he's cynical when he believes he's being realistic.
- She doesn't want to be called childlike and ignorant when she tries to express her optimistic views of life.
- He doesn't want to be told he fears closeness when he believes he's been giving his all to the relationship in every way he knows how.
- She doesn't want to be told she's engulfing when she believes she is simply trying to bring them closer together and to have the relationship survive in the face of his withdrawal.
- He doesn't want to be accused of being cold

and unfeeling when he is trying to be objective and reasonable.

- She doesn't want to be called irrational or impossible when she is talking in a heartfelt way rather than coldly and objectively.
- He doesn't want to be accused of trying to control when he sees himself simply as taking responsibility for what, if left to her, he feels wouldn't be done properly or promptly, because of her lack of "awareness" about the world.
- She becomes irritated when she's told that she's indecisive when she feels she really needs to think carefully and not rush into making a decision.
- He doesn't want to be accused of not doing enough as a father when, as the primary provider for the family, he feels he's giving his fair share as a parent.
- She doesn't want to be told that she is too involved as a mother and is hurting her children by being overprotective, when she sees herself simply as loving them and making their needs a priority.

And so the cycle goes, until the wounds and miscommunications, and feelings of futility become overwhelming and the bond breaks. In summary, because of the opposing experience of the same realities, the loving intentions on both sides are viewed exactly the opposite of the way they are intended. When each person believes they are giving everything, they soon discover that they are being experienced by their partner as selfish, neurotic, or uncaring.

Without a mutual empathy and compassion for

the reality of each partner, a sense of hopelessness and "giving up" is inevitable, together with a feeling of being trapped by the other as each grows tired of explaining and justifying and feeling unappreciated and misunderstood.

Who's Using Whom? Men and Women as Objects/Men and Women as People

A well-known female celebrity, famed for her ability to attract wealthy and powerful men, gave the following advice to her single friends: "The first time you marry for love. The second time for security. The last time you get married, it should be for companionship."

Unknowingly, she was verbalizing a philosophy on the best uses of a man at different stages of a woman's life. It is not much different from the many books written to teach women how to get and hold a good man.

Another woman talking about the man she would like to marry stressed the necessity of his having a good economic future and of being the type of person who would be a responsible, involved father. Although her standards were certainly understandable, without realizing it she was describing men as objects to fulfill a function, not as people. She didn't mention personal qualities but described instead a man's ability "to perform."

Women may not consider that as a form of

using, but many men today interpret it that way. Listen to Tom, who described it as follows.

"I know I'm being used because when I stop 'doing for' a woman and just talk about my feelings or preoccupations, I notice that most of the time they're not really interested, or that they even get annoyed at my 'lack of depth and sensitivity.' They want to talk about the relationship. That's all that seems important.

"So long as I'm doing what I'm supposed to, I'm lovable. I don't mind being useful because I need that myself. But I want to feel that when I'm not performing, I also have some value. It reminds me of my childhood when my father continually implied I was worthless unless I was doing something."

It is easy enough to see the "sexism" of one's partner—the feeling of being used to perform services, without seeing how we do the same thing in a different way. Each partner can justify his or her own sexism, while feeling abused by the sexism of the other.

In their angry, "lucid" moments each sex comes to feel they've been "had"—yet can rarely recognize their own part in the mutual using process.

Traditional men are unintentional sexists because everything personal is kept at arm's length and all relationships are viewed in terms of goals and purposes rather than in terms of closeness and caring.

Women are unintentional sexists when men are experienced as "sexy" because they are ambitious or successful. The symbols of material achievement in the world make him attractive to her just as her symbols of beauty make her attractive to him. In both cases, the inner person is not being considered.

Fear and loathing about being used as an object lie just below the surface for both sexes even in the most romantic of beginnings. The "gut level" response that the other person sees more than is really there, and one can't be fully honest for fear of losing the magic, is realistic. Neither is being seen or fully accepted as they know themselves to be. Images are projected and that image is being loved. When the person behind the image emerges later, anger and disappointment occur. The other person is accused of pretending to be something they really weren't.

Women can identify their own sexism through the following reactions:

1. When a man does something perceived as hurtful, and her reaction is, "He's just like a man!"
2. When upon first meeting a man, what he does for a living and how successfully he does it are the major factors determining whether he's seen as desirable and interesting. A lesser status occupation makes him less desirable and attractive.
3. When a man who is supposedly "special" and "loved" is reluctant to commit, he is abandoned.
4. When a man agrees to be open and honest and then reveals his feelings, he is accused of being hurtful and insensitive.
5. When a man is seen as desirable because he's believed to be "different from other men," meaning men are seen as a negative stereotype and not as people.

When two objects get together, there is resistance to *knowing* the other person as they know themselves to be, much like the disinterest in knowing personally someone we hire to work for us. When a person is loved—not the function—conflict and differences are rarely serious enough to do real damage, and the emphasis is on our feelings rather than on what the other person can do for us.

The "state of the art" of relationships traditionally has been for men and women to choose each other based on symbols and function; how we can be enhanced or rescued by them, which is disguised behind a cloak of "intimacy."

In recent years, women's and men's anger toward each other has come from the growing awareness of being used by the opposite sex. Such insights, however, have not been coupled with the awareness that using is what *both* sexes traditionally have been taught to do. A search for ways to transform relationships into caring friendships is the real struggle for both. Mutual accusation can only bring a distorted sense of wariness and distrust, and a self-righteous sense of being wounded and vulnerable.

Triggering Each Other: How the Dance Is Done

1. His guilt, coming from a defensively exaggerated sense of his power and responsibility, is met by her blaming, stemming

from a defensive repression and denial of her power.

2. This process produces an undue sense of being hurtful in him, in tandem with a defensive sense of being the innocent and loving "victim" in her.
3. His defensively inflated ego causes him to feel more powerful in the relationship than he actually is ("It'll crush her if I'm honest with her"). This is counterpart to a defensively diminished, vulnerable, or dissolved ego or a low sense of self-esteem and power in her, causing her to feel taken for granted and not really needed.
4. His interpretation of their interaction is based on what he can see or measure objectively outside of himself, and goes along with her internalization or interpretation of events based on inner feelings.
5. His resistance to talking about "us" exists together with her preoccupation with the relationship, and her apparent "inability to stop" focusing on it.
6. His defensive anger and aggression coupled with his tendency to deny his vulnerability are counterpart to her tendency to deny conflict, an inability to acknowledge anger, and a desire to avoid conflict.
7. A woman's resistance to or denial of her power to take control occurs along with experiencing herself as controlled and a resentment of the man for his desire to control. This is counterpart to a man's need to control, believing that he is omnipotent and that she needs his guidance.

This makes him feel guilty and responsible when things go wrong.

8. His lack of feelings and insensitivity and the tendency to approach relationships objectively, believing that personal matters can be conducted by using logic, are counterpart to her tendency to show emotion and to be unduly sensitive to what he says and does because she is emotionally overinvolved.
9. Her longing for romance and a positive view of life and her fantasy of having a close, intimate relationship are counterpart to his tendency to be cautious about love, to view romance as unrealistic, and to view the world as dangerous, and thus to be wary and resistant to getting too deeply involved in the relationship lest he lose his focus on the "dangers" out there. She sees that as a resistance to closeness with her and the intimacy she needs, and he considers her demands for intimacy as part of her childlike naïveté.
10. Her tendency to get too close and to seek an intimacy that is really a fusion of two people into one, triggers his tendency to get "too distant," to become fixated on issues of freedom and autonomy.
11. She has a tendency to say, "Men are just like *that*" and to feel distressed by what he does, as if he is doing it intentionally to hurt her, without seeing how her responses impact him and increase his tendency to feel "that's how women are," without being able to recognize behaviors

that polarize him and "drive him up the wall."

12. His gender undertow emerges on the surface and expresses itself in him through his speeches about freedom, space, and autonomy, and in her by lectures on commitment, closeness, and love.
13. He talks sexual excitement because he requires external stimulation. This need created his initial attraction and sexual fantasy. Conversely, she needs romantic emotion and close, personal intensity for fulfilling sexuality. This makes her vulnerable to those who speak eloquently and manipulatively of love and relationships as a priority of life, such as poets, therapists, gurus, clergy, and professors.
14. He believes that by talking reasonably and being logical, the relationship will improve. He can't see how this logic triggers feelings in her of being distanced and rejected. She responds more emotionally in the desire to reach him and make him more sensitive to bring them closer, which pushes him away still more, causing him to become even more detached in his responses.
15. When they talk of the world outside themselves, their different visions of the world become obvious. He sees the world as a chaotic place, because he views it from the vantage point of self-protective needs for control, separateness, and power. She sees the "dawn of a new age," a world heading toward universal love, spirituality, and peace—free of barriers and boundaries

and filled with people who care for each other.

So the dance of polarization goes. The more extreme these opposing experiences, the greater the pain, frustration, and sense of futility that makes escape the only way to save oneself and not feel overwhelmed by a relationship of increasing pain.

Don't Blame Him! Don't Blame Yourself!

In our personal relationships, we get what the mutually triggering process creates—with both sexes being unknowing perpetrators and both being victims because of the inability to acknowledge their own defensive response. Denial exists in both sexes equally, just as does the desire to love.

Blaming and vindicating oneself or feeling guilty and hating oneself are results of a distorted perception of this shared struggle. It underscores the inability to understand the *fully mutual triggering process.* Until shared struggles and polarized realities can be acknowledged by each sex and worked through in tandem, the fragile bond between the sexes can only become more fragile, and neither is really to blame.

6

Making Him Over: What to Know Before You Try

Natalie, a woman of thirty-four, who was stuck in an unfulfilling marriage, heard her husband describe his idea of being loved as "being left alone until I feel ready to talk or be affectionate, and not to be blamed for feeling that way."

Natalie's initial reaction was to feel angry and rejected. She thought to herself, "What a self-centered jerk! How can I have a relationship with—much less love—a man who tells me to leave him alone until *he's ready*. How could I be such a masochist?"

Having promised herself to be patient, however, and to try to see things from his perspective and experience, she did not give in to this initial feeling. Instead, she tried to understand why he felt this way, yet still claim to love her and to want to be with her. The two sounded incompatible. She remembered, however, the many times before she got married, when she would say essentially the same thing to men she liked but whom she didn't want to go to bed with; men who pressured her for sex before she felt ready. "Leave me alone until I feel ready—and don't make me feel guilty about it," she remembered telling them. The men who were able to accept that message without criticism and who respected her wishes were those with whom she eventually came to feel close and sexually responsive.

Natalie was happily surprised when the closer she came to hearing and accepting her husband's need for time and distance, without taking it personally as a rejection, the more she began to receive the kinds of closeness and intimacy from him that she wanted.

Similarly, Joanna is a woman who had been in a relationship with a man for nine years—a man who continually found reasons to postpone marriage. In her frustration she sought counseling and in her sessions began to understand how her urgency to marry, and the fact that commitment was constantly on her mind, dominated the relationship's atmosphere, obscured the positive, happy elements of it, and caused her partner to doubt her love. In other words, her emphasis on marriage was creating the opposite effect from what she intended.

When she finally could say to herself, "I don't want to marry a man who's not ready to marry me, but I love being with him so I'll continue to spend time with him," and acted accordingly, things changed. She continued her relationship but also began to date another man who did wish to marry her.

Rather than use that as a weapon to pressure or intimidate her boyfriend, she simply told him that since he wasn't sure he wanted to marry her and because marriage was important to her, she intended to focus more on the other relationship. Her boyfriend's response to her changed radically when it became clear that marriage was no longer her dominant preoccupation in spending time with him, and that he might lose the companionship and warmth that he cherished.

When asked about his turnabout, he replied. "When I no longer felt a pressure to marry, I trusted Joanna's love and affection more. It reassured me that she wasn't using me simply to get her needs met, but that she spent time with me because she really liked me. That seemed to free me to trust her fully. Once that was behind me, I discovered I really *wanted* to marry her." However, now Joanna resisted because she wasn't sure anymore. "I love being around you, but I feel you want to get married because you don't want the other guy to have me. I don't want a wedding based on that."

"By the time she said yes, Joanna had regained the power and self-respect she had when we first met—and then had lost in her urgency to marry. Joanna was secure and relaxed again and we were able to enjoy the relationship like never before. By the time of our wedding, our desire to marry, I believe, was truly equal."

Based on twenty-five years' experience intensively counseling hundreds of men, I can safely say that the attempt to change a man is difficult under the best of conditions, even when his motivation is high. The strictures of his conditioning make him fearful of giving up control, and being vulnerable. Approaching a relationship with an expectation that he will change is not only futile, but achieves the opposite effect. It increases his defensiveness, rigidity, distrust, and resistance. The change occurs only after a foundation of trust and safety is built.

Although a man may make cosmetic changes under pressure out of guilt or the desire to be a "nice guy," accusing him of being selfish and fearing closeness, and then persisting in discussing his relationship problems, alienates him.

Men in relationships believe that they are caring and open to love. They are bewildered when that belief is challenged. One man explained this feeling: "She says she loves me and wants to be closer but it doesn't feel that way to me. The message I get from her about the way I relate is that I don't do it right and there's something damaged about me. If that's actually so, why does she want to even be close to me? If a woman doesn't basically think I'm okay, I can't believe her when she says she cares."

Approaching Him for Change

The foundation for change in a relationship has to be built in part through a man's experience of it, not from the vantage point of a woman's needs for intimacy and love, in order for the change to be effective and lasting. If a man's expressed "reality" in the relationship then turns out to be offensive to a woman (which may be the case in some relationships), at least it frees her to back away from an intense pursuit of intimacy and reassess the nature of her own feelings of love and involvement. "Maybe I don't love him like I think I do, and maybe I should have some serious reservations about the degree of my involvement," is how one women expressed it upon reflection.

By listening to and understanding a man's

experience of a relationship, he gets a sense that his partner is actually relating to *him* as a person, not just as an object to satisfy her needs.

It is my belief that when men "tune out" or seem preoccupied when spoken to, it is partially because what is being said to them is not related to what they experience in the relationship. Thus the words he hears sound to him like a self-serving monologue. On some level he "knows" that his partner is not really talking to him, but to a fantasy projection created by her needs. His loss of concentration reflects that subliminal awareness, even if he is not able to understand and articulate what it is he's responding to consciously.

Using the notion of a man's reality as a starting point, the following are three background "secrets" of approaching men for change in a relationship.

1. *You can't "love" a man into changing.*

In fact, the opposite is more likely to occur. Men seem most willing and able to make changes when they get the message, by virtue of a woman's self-esteem that if he doesn't pay close attention to who she is, and what her needs are, she will pull away, not to punish him but to seek fulfillment for herself.

What many women seem to believe is a loving attitude designed to help a man change is not experienced that way at all. Her "love" is experienced as neediness that generates his guilt about the inability to give her what she wants. Also, he may perceive her motives as selfish. He feels pressured, not loved, and thus he pulls inward.

The notion that most men are wounded little

boys at heart, who need to be loved in order to be "healed," may be partially true. But, as with wounded animals, a distrustful and self-protective reaction occurs toward someone coming too close too fast.

2. *Changing a man has more to do with how a woman feels about herself than what she does in the relationship.*

"I trust a woman who likes herself and has a satisfying life she is committed to," is how it was expressed by one man. It is *how* a woman relates to a man, and the degree of personal esteem and autonomy she communicates, that will "change him" in a trusting, loving way.

A woman's inner security allows her to back away when appropriate, without pressure, anger, or anxiety. Then her loving of a man becomes a realistic response to the way he *is*, whereas strategies to change him fail because he senses them as being manipulative and self-serving. It is that aspect, I believe, that causes him to withdraw and avoid closeness.

3. *The most effective way to change a man is to identify and change the response or behavior that triggers his undesirable response.*

A woman who wants closeness with a man needs to focus on what she does to push him away rather than on "his problem" with intimacy.

The woman who feels controlled needs to focus on what she does to give away power, not on the man's controlling behavior.

The woman who feels he is treating her like a child needs to focus on ways she is promoting that response through expressions of helplessness or clinging behavior, not by confrontation of his chauvinism.

The woman who "loves too much" needs to focus on her overly intense involvement in a one-way relationship rather than on his "selfish" ways.

The woman whose partner becomes silent and withdrawn needs to learn what triggers this silence rather than trying to coax him into opening up.

Although men do not change readily, women in relationships have great power to bring out the best or worst of a man's behaviors. Most men can become Prince Charming or Mr. Rat, depending on how they are approached. When a woman relates to a man on the basis of his experience and reality of a relationship, his best traits will tend to emerge. When she has to relate to him on that basis, it also tests the substance of her loving. However, if a woman's motivation to change a man is subjective, based on hurt feelings and frustration, his worst defensive traits will emerge.

The most productive effort for a woman seeking change is to remain the strong, non-judgmental, independent, and assertive "best person" that she really is—with or without him. One man expressed it as, "I loved her for the way she was in the world and with people when I met her. She was direct, playful, funny, and relaxed. Now when she relates to me and the relationship she's almost one hundred and eighty degrees opposite to those things. She's vague, tense, serious, and easily brought to tears. *That* is driving me away."

The frustrating element here is that most women do return to being their "best self," but only after they end a relationship. A thirty-five-year-old, highly successful businesswoman was involved with a man who had become completely cold and detached, partially in reaction to the fact that she had lost her ability to relate to him in a direct and objective fashion. Instead, when they were together she was fearful, cried easily, and unable to express her needs clearly. By the time the relationship was on the verge of collapse, no abuse on his part, such as stony silence or disappearance for days to be with a lover whom he blatantly lied to her about, could get her to respond in a strong and forceful manner.

Almost immediately after they broke up, however, she became a totally different person. Actually, she became the confident, assertive, and humorous person her friends knew her to be. She became involved with another man, and her behavior with him was radically different than it had been with her ex-husband.

Alienating Approaches to Change: How to Guarantee Failure

1. *Make him feel guilty.*

Typical assertions that alienate men include: "You're so nice to everyone else, and I have to catch your negativity and bad moods"; or "Every time you treat me this way, I can't do my work, or concentrate on anything because I'm so upset"; "Everything is a priority in your life except me."

Although guilt may sometimes induce surface change, it creates an undertow of anger and increased "pulling away" and resistance to closeness in him.

2. *Confront him about his relationship inadequacies.*

Commonly expressed alienating assertions include, "You're selfish and insensitive and only interested in taking care of number one"; "You don't know what love is. All you know is how to take"; "I have to pay the price because you can't stand your mother"; or, "You've never learned how to give to someone."

Men do have relationship deficiencies, and they hear about them constantly. Being confronted about their "deficits" only drives them further away.

3. *Interpret his behavior negatively.*

"You're afraid of intimacy"; "You don't want anybody to get close to you"; "You hate women"; and "You're paying me back for what your mother did to you."

Even when these interpretations are accurate, they are equal in impact to a man's interpretations of the woman's behavior to explain relationship problems, as follows: "You hate men"; "You want to be taken care of like your dad did for your mom"; "You want me to play perfect daddy"; or "Your love and niceness are a cover-up for your anger."

Both sexes have unresolved issues about each

other and troublesome motivations in relationships. Although intended to be helpful, however, negative interpretations are likely to be experienced as an attack and a form of rejection and criticism, or as self-serving manipulations.

4. *Continue to talk to him about the relationship when he's hit an overload and asked you to stop.*

Many men feel about relationship talk the way most women feel about sports or business talk—a little goes a long way. To him, the themes and observations in relationship talk tend to become repetitive, boring, and irritating, just as men's talk about mechanics or politics does.

The real message conveyed by a woman's persistence in discussing the relationship is "Let's talk about why you're not more involved, why you won't open up, or what's wrong with you, and why you're incapable of relating intimately." Pursuing such discussions promotes withdrawal and negative reactions.

Because most men's primary focus in life tends to be external, they may tend to lose interest in personal discussion sooner than women. Being insensitive to this tendency and reacting in a negative way creates further "closing up."

5. *Compare him to other men.*

"Look at the way your friend Ted treats his wife. There's such respect and love for her. You're the only one of your friends who doesn't seem to care about involving himself with his wife and family."

He doesn't believe this is true. Behind the seemingly different veneers, the conflicts and resistances experienced by men in relationships are similar, and he knows that. Comparing him with others convinces him that the woman is naïve in her observations and is unduly critical and unsupportive. To him, the observations reflect her disappointment to him as a person and her resentment, and are more likely construed as a hostile attack than as a constructive effort to generate closeness.

In general, pressuring a man to change through accusation, blame, comparison with others, and guilt-inducing expressions of sadness and pain about the relationship may produce superficial change. However, the longer-range price for changes based on the assumption that he is the spoiler is that his connection to the relationship is destroyed. Any change that results from confronting him with negative feedback about himself is change by his further emotional withdrawal and a buildup of frustration in the woman, who believes he is deliberately acting in selfish ways, which are the cornerstones for the ultimate deterioration of the relationship.

How to Distinguish Real Change from the Surface Appearance of Change

Authentic change in relationships occurs when both partners become aware of their own contributions to the problem, accompanied by the willingness and capacity to acknowledge and work at changing themselves. When superficial change has taken place, the old patterns are destined to reappear.

For example, many women have trouble recognizing and communicating their anger in a direct way. They are distressed and want to avoid "negative" exchanges. This resistance is comparable to men's inability to recognize and express personal needs and vulnerability. Thus, interaction between men and women is damaged when men tend to become cold, withdrawn, and angry because they can't communicate their vulnerability, or when women cry, accuse, or act injured instead of directly expressing their anger. Lasting change in a relationship is realized when both partners recognize their own problem areas and are able to express themselves fully, directly, and honestly in order to change a relationship pattern, instead of responding defensively and emotionally.

False change involves "trying" but failing to come to grips with that which each partner has difficulty expressing. So he walks on eggshells, fearful of making her angry, and she urgently anticipates all his needs and vulnerability, and thereby assumes a mothering role so that he never has to express himself directly or acknowledge these problems within himself. Such "sensitivity" to each other produces short-lived changes and temporary sentimental promises to make things better. The changes, however, have no roots based on the real causes, so they fail to survive.

Solutions and change that involve avoidance of each other's hot buttons tend to make things worse because hopelessness builds in each partner when they come to believe they have really tried and "it didn't help."

"How-To" Strategies As Avoidance of Change

A common effort at achieving change, and one that will prove futile, is what I call "change by external strategy," or "how to." This involves doing something that is done for effect, but is insincere. It is an approach that is always guaranteed to fail—like diet and exercise programs that don't address the deeper aspects underlying the problem. It is what makes and keeps authors and publishers of panacea books wealthy.

Anna was a woman addicted to a man she described as "cold and selfish." In her support group she was told that men abuse women who makes themselves too available, and only become interested when a woman plays "hard to get."

Even though she felt an urgent need for reassurance from her boyfriend, she began to pretend indifference. After a few such efforts, her partner began to pay more attention and show greater interest and affection. Because she had not come to terms with the deeper aspects of her problem, however, unknowingly she built up such an intense neediness that as soon as he became more interested and involved, she responded with such great urgency that he pulled away once again. Now more than ever he saw her as inconsistent, unpredictable, and "crazy" because of her extreme, irrational shifts. Anna was left with a greater sense of despair than before—an attitude that "Nothing works with him. I give up."

How-to strategies are essentially manipulations and therefore create greater distrust and self-protective distance. Although they may produce short-term changes, these changes serve to create a deepening sense of hopelessness because they focus on one person's problems, and not the relationship dynamics.

Fallacies of Change

Surface appearances aside, in a relationship where two people chose each other because they were strongly attracted, the deterioration of the relationship is a two-way process, a cycle in which each participates in pushing the other away in tandem by triggering the other partner's most defensive tendencies. Unless both partners, in search of healing their relationship, focus on themselves, lasting change is impossible.

A major obstacle to change is the tendency to identify an external cause or reason. Common ones include, "He works too much," "She's let herself go," "He's always watching sports," "She's obsessed with soap operas and food," "He's not affectionate," "She's insecure," and so on. While these may create temporary reassurance that the cause is external, the real work of change and growth is undermined.

The following fallacious notions about change damage the relationship.

1. One partner really cares and knows how to be loving, whereas the other one doesn't.
2. One person is primarily to blame for the problems in the relationship, whereas the other is the healthy or the good one, valiantly working to keep things going.
3. One partner is caring; the other is hostile.

These notions and approach to change create the kinds of polarization guaranteed to turn the relationship into a finger-pointing nightmare.

In the power struggle for intimacy, each sets out to make the other person feel responsible for the pain and problems of the relationship and sees themselves as the patient and loving partner. Women blame men's coldness; men blame women's emotionalizing. Men blame women's nagging and women blame men's refusal to open up. Women blame men's anger and critical nature, men blame women's hypersensitivity. Women blame men's compulsive need to work, and men blame women's passivity and lack of direction. So it goes in the game of blame until the weight of negativity finally destroys the relationship.

On the Woman's Side:

From my experience as a psychotherapist, *the single greatest obstacle* to change and the development of genuine intimacy in women is the sense of being an injured, loving partner in a relationship with a selfish, nonloving mate. That interpretation of a relationship develops in women as an unconscious by-product of the process by which traditional relationships begin and then develop. This sense of injury is a product of the deeper undercurrents that are building while love is first blooming. It includes:

1. Romantic relating, where women tend to be *reactors* to men. This generates a sense of feeling controlled, powerless, taken for granted, and with losing their identity in the relationship. Waiting for the man to initiate dating, take responsibility for the decisions on a date while trying to be agreeable, is the very same process that initially sparks most traditional relationships and at the same time lays the groundwork for the woman's injured feelings.
2. The tendency to accommodate and adapt to a man's preferences, schedule, lifestyle, and social interests. This accommodation is the traditional feminine role of the giver, who then comes to feel taken for granted, discounted, used, or treated as a nobody.
3. Placing a disproportionate emphasis on the relationship at the expense of other aspects of one's life. This tends to make a woman overly sensitive to the most minute aspects of the interaction. Also, because few men are as relationship focused as women, women tend to become resentful, feeling that they are giving much more than they are getting, so the man is seen as selfish and disinterested.
4. The tendency to seek a closeness with her partner that he is incapable of giving and then, out of the insecurity generated by a feeling of "He doesn't really care," seeking continual reas-

surance. This generates a self-protective, defensive response in the man, who reacts negatively to the feelings of being smothered and drained by the pressure to prove his love. When he responds with irritation, it is interpreted falsely as his rejecting a woman's caring and trying to show love.

Friends who can see only the superficial aspects of the relationship on the surface, may confirm the woman's belief that she is involved with a man who can't love. Even he may begin to feel there is something wrong with him, that he is inferior and insensitive because he can't respond positively to a woman's loving intensity. Such feedback undermines the potential for a better balance by placing the responsibility on only one partner.

The man can't change in the relationship by himself, no matter how much he tries. Nor can he change until his partner becomes aware of her impact on him and of her role in creating the tensions that accompany the relationship.

To the extent that the relationship is interpreted as loving partner (her) and selfish, unloving partner (him), lasting change in the man and within the relationship becomes impossible.

On the other hand, depending on the extent to which a woman can recognize her impact on the relationship and the reciprocity of the accompanying problems, a relationship can be repaired and brought to its best potential fairly easily. It requires only the ability and willingness to map the problem correctly so that distortions that make one partner seem hurtful and the other blameless, can be identified and changed.

As a therapist, my diagnostic rule of thumb is

as follows: To the degree that one partner sees the other as the cause of the relationship's problems, change is slowed. When one partner sees him or herself as blameless, change is impossible. When both partners focus on their own impact on the process they want to change to improve the relationship, change can occur readily and love can once again dominate.

Changing Him by Understanding Your Impact: The Specifics

The following are responses in women that tend to polarize men.

1. Intense emotionalizing has the same negative effect on a man, and produces the same anger in him, that his cold, analytical, and detached attitude triggers in a woman.
2. Blaming a man for the problems of the relationship, which reinforces his sense of self-hatred and futility and his feelings of being misunderstood. It also promotes a need to escape and seek validation with a new partner.
3. Pressuring for closeness and asking to be held in the midst of an angry confrontation acts as a double assault on a man's sensibilities. He is being made to feel guilty about his need for distance at the very time that

he is feeling least capable of showing affection.

4. Being critical of his "doing" approach to the relationship, which discounts the validity of his way of loving. Negating "doing" as "not real love" is tantamount to rejection, and it will drive him away.
5. Accusing him of disliking or fearing women and closeness, which will make him feel falsely accused. He thinks that he does love his partner and that he is fond of women.
6. Perceiving him as being insincere when he attempts to change because his efforts seem forced and deliberate. Men's efforts may seem mechanical and false because they are premeditated rather than felt. Without inner change, this is the way men try.
7. Assertions that he acts hurtful and rejecting because he doesn't care, which will generate a sense of futility in him and the desire to stop trying.

The following will bring him closer.

1. Inviting him to express his experience of the relationship and using that as a guide for gauging the psychological distance between the two partners and the changes that need to be made. This will give him a positive feeling about the relationship and generate a willingness to try to change it.
2. Asking him for specifics regarding what you do to upset him, and attempting to change. This will reassure him that his experience is acknowledged and validated.
3. Waiting for *him* to reach out without pres-

suring him for closeness. This is the *quickest* way to bring him out of himself.
4. A reduced emphasis on the relationship and more emphasis on externals and the kinds of things that interest him, because a true change in him toward the personal and away from impersonal goals and achievements will generate initial anxiety, fear, and resistance, and must be approached with caution.

Knowing When Not to Try for Change: Indications of a Poisoned Relationship

Relationships can reach a point where mutual growth within them is almost impossible and, for the sake of both partners, serious consideration should be given to ending the relationship. When a number of the following situations exist, the unconscious polarization process has deeply poisoned the relationship.

1. There is violence or the constant threat of a violent eruption, regardless of who is to blame.
2. "Innocent" comments and unintended slights or acts escalate rapidly into angry outbursts, coldness, and alienation that lasts for days.
3. Both partners' lives are dominated by addictive "escape" behaviors, such as

compulsive eating, working, TV watching, drinking, drugs, and there is very little affectionate, personal contact.

4. "Death wishes" toward a partner dominate one's fantasy life. These are feelings that death by accident or illness would be a welcome liberation from the relationship and the easiest solution.
5. Being together is enervating. There is boredom and disinterest whenever these partners are alone, with no external activity to distract them.
6. The times apart are the "holidays" one looks forward to, whereas the times spent together are dreaded.
7. The sole way to be comfortably together is via distraction, such as watching videos, going out to eat, or engaging in activities that discourage close interaction.
8. Feeling that you are "dying" in the relationship, or you don't care if you do, because you are chronically depressed.
9. When in bed at night, your body tenses up and you seek to avoid physical contact with your partner.
10. On weekend mornings, you get out of bed as early as possible to avoid any sustained intimate involvement.
11. It is almost impossible to listen to your partner without becoming distracted or irritated by what is said or how it is stated.
12. The habits and mannerisms of your partner annoy or disgust you.

A Final Note on Traditional Advice on How to Change or Excite Your Partner

The unhappiness women experience when their relationship is threatened may cause them unknowingly to do the opposite of what is effective and what is necessary to improve it.

When men are "turned off" sexually or personally, and they seem bored or withdrawn, they've reached a personal overload. Much like an electrical circuit, the psychological breakers of his deeper self have caused a shutdown of his system. Traditional advice on how to promote closeness by luring him back into involvement, sexually or otherwise, is like forcing additional electric current through an already overloaded system.

Remember when your partner was most readily connected to the relationship and no effort was required to excite him? That was probably during the earliest stages of the relationship, when distance and the stimulation of newness and a controllable separateness were present. His "system" was open.

Were it not for a woman's underlying anxieties that create a tendency for overreaction and the need for reassurance, it would be apparent what she should do when a man withdraws, and she would do it readily.

Pursuing him with "techniques" designed to excite him may be correct in content, but are ineffective and counterproductive in process, and it is the process or *how* of the relationship that creates its energy and involvement level, and not the *what*, or external content.

7

Relating to Him Realistically: An Overview

The Basic Realities: Starting Points for a Mutual Intimacy

1. *A traditional man cannot completely fulfill a traditional woman's needs. Therefore, the more intense her needs for closeness, reassurance, security, or fulfillment, the greater the anger and frustration that will develop over his supposed selfishness, insensitivity, and his inability to be close. Similarly, anger will build in him for being held responsible and blamed for something he feels is unfair and untrue.*

Just as no woman can satisfy a man's need to "feel like a man" and to fill the bottomless-well compulsion to validate his masculinity, women's intimacy needs are equally as unfillable and men who try inevitably fail.

When a woman's intimacy needs are particularly intense, the needs serve to push him even further away. They polarize him in defensive counterreaction to move still further outside of himself. He becomes more compelled to control his sense of pressure and the desire to get away. Finally he becomes the stereotype of a detached, cold, insensitive man—an end point that is beyond his conscious control or intention.

The notion that men intentionally frustrate women or withhold themselves out of selfishness is a cornerstone distortion that promotes the breakdown of the fragile developing love bond between the sexes. The unmet needs and expectations for intimacy create ongoing conflict. Each partner feels misunderstood and provoked by the other.

Relating to men realistically means knowing what needs they can and cannot fulfill; what needs stem from feminine insecurity; and how relationship pressures on a man polarize him and trigger his defensive relationship behaviors.

2. *Men do not hurt women intentionally.*

It is the out-of-control mutually polarizing dynamic that transforms initially intense romantic love, euphoria, desire, and sensitivity into hostility and what seems to be selfish, abusive behavior but is actually only a defensive counterreaction. Just as women find themselves turning on a man in anger because they feel their needs are being intentionally frustrated, so men become abusive in their ineffectual response to demands and pressures they can't respond to and that provoke them.

Only those seeking to create a scapegoat for a complex and unconsciously defensive interactional problem would propose and promote the perception and belief that men commit to women and marry and derive pleasure and fulfillment from being self-centered and abusive. Equally as damaging is the notion that men could, if they so desired, be what the woman wanted them to be. Such interpretations are erroneous and the death knell of mutual growth and genuine intimacy between the sexes. As long as men's motives and behavior are interpreted negatively, movement toward a healthy mutual caring and love cannot occur.

Being in a relationship should be a tacit acknowledgment that men, like women, do their conscious best to make their central relationship work. Men bring their own intense needs for love and fulfillment to the relationship, and whatever negative behaviors they exhibit are the result of the polarization that evolves in the relationship. The process leaves them equally as despairing and frustrated as their partner.

Relating to a man realistically means acknowledging that men do not enter love relationships with an intention or desire to be hurtful and that abusive behavior is a symptom of a sick relationship, not of a selfish, destructive man.

3. *Men cannot make women feel good about themselves in a relationship.*

A woman with low self-esteem will eventually experience her partner as being critical, unsupportive, and unappreciative of her worth and contributions to their relationship. These feelings are a product of a woman's deeper anxieties about her self-worth, and the negative response that this promotes in men who feel pressured to reassure her that they appreciate and love her.

4. *Men show love and caring the way they have*

been taught to. What they don't show, they can't show or never learned.

Men express love and intimacy primarily by "doing for" rather than by the expression of emotion and personal closeness. This way of expressing love is as crucial to the existence and survival of the relationship as is a woman's focus on emotional closeness. Men experience themselves as being loving when they are "doing for" and taking responsibility and the initiative through action. Men are polarized when these expressions of love are seen as forms of avoiding closeness.

Relating to a man realistically therefore means acknowledging that although his love is expressed differently than a woman's, it is no less meaningful, real, or intense.

5. *A man's masculine socialization externalizes him and focuses him on performance and achievement matters.*

Men's personal insensitivities are the result of this repression and closing off of their inner selves. Their sensibilities, feelings, needs, and vulnerabilities are blocked in the process of becoming a man. The masculine ideal is personified by the man who is goal directed, analytic, self-contained, aggressive, unemotional, and personally invulnerable.

Relating to men realistically means recognizing that their sensitivities are focused externally and that the ways men show insensitivity are the direct result of this blocked development of their personal self.

The combination of a woman's need for closeness and intimacy and a man's externalization, if not acknowledged and mutually corrected, is the basic reason for the pain and suffering that evolve in relationships.

6. *Under conditions of relationship stress, such as during arguments and conflicts, men tend to disconnect in a heightened direction of externalized defensiveness or detachment. This is their form of self-protection. The greater pressure or stress that they experience in the relationship, the more extreme is this tendency to disconnect, causing them to seem distant, uncaring, and cold. Contrariwise, when he feels unpressured and safe, he becomes capable of being warm and responsive once again.*

It is counterproductive and dangerously provocative to pressure a man to get closer and to open up during those times when he is being pulled in the other direction. It tends to polarize him even more and to produce greater disconnection.

Relating to men realistically means recognizing this inevitable disconnection, when men experience an overload of personal stress. As the stress lessens, men "bounce back." A woman's urgent need for closeness as a man withdraws, escalates the tensions, widens the intimacy gap, and makes the relationship seem hopeless.

7. *To love a man realistically requires being aware of how he experiences the relationship and the love that a woman gives him, not rejecting or reacting critically and punitively upon hearing him articulate this experience.*

Relating to men realistically requires acknowledgment that a man's experience of a woman's love and caring are different from a woman's. To love a man truly means generating an atmosphere that makes it safe and welcoming for him to "open up" about this experience. No real closeness can occur without such an awareness and acceptance of that difference.

8. *A woman's intense personal focus and the giving herself over to the relationship, at the expense of her separate identity and boundaries, is damaging and polarizing. It causes women to see themselves as giving and loving more than the man, and it causes him to be perceived as self-centered and unappreciative of her love.*

Men are at their loving best when stimulated and challenged by a woman who does not accommodate and "sacrifice" herself to the relationship even though a man may complain when a woman does not make herself readily available, or fails to make his needs her central focus. This is part of the unconscious testing process and power struggle of a relationship. Although men may "try" to control their partner, men respond badly if they succeed.

Similarly, women who are uncomfortable taking control or power may unconsciously give it over to the man, and then resent him when this happens.

Men lose interest in the women who lose their identities in a relationship, but remain connected to and stimulated by the woman who keeps her boundaries and maintains a strong, separate identity.

Relating to men realistically means recognizing that a woman's intense relationship involvement and focus is self-destructive and destructive to the relationship. Her "self-sacrifice" to the relationship is an unconscious compulsion that is not experienced as love by the man, which is why it produces a negative and abusive response from him.

9. *Men are not dangerous to women; sick or polarized relationships are.*

As relationships polarize—a process triggered by and participated in equally and unknowingly by both partners—men become cold, disconnected, critical, and abusive because of the tension that builds up on their end of the imbalance. These same men in a nonpolarized or balanced relationship can be deeply loving, gentle, and sensitive.

The polarizing process makes men behave in hurtful and destructive ways, and it is this process, unconsciously created by a mutual triggering of defensive responses, and not male chauvinism, that endangers women in committed relationships.

In fully polarized interactions, men and women interact in their "sickest," most defensively hostile ways. As that polarization is eased, men are once again able to express love.

Relating to men realistically means understanding that hurtful behaviors are not inherent in male sexism but are a by-product of the process of unconscious, mutual triggering and polarization, which can only be changed by the participation of both.

10. *Although men may not be able to articulate it, their need for the central man-woman relationship is at least as strong as their partner's*

because of men's personal, emotional isolation and the personal deprivation that develops in their lives as a result of their conditioning.

Relating to men realistically means recognizing that men's dependency on and need for love and the relationship they are in may not be as clearly expressed as a woman's but is intense nevertheless. Once involved in a relationship, he attaches strongly to it and becomes extremely dependent on it.

11. *Authentic love between a man and woman, given the powerful experiential differences between the sexes, builds slowly by dealing with the significant conflicts that inevitably arise.*

A woman's equation between love and "being nice" or "getting along" without fights and anger is fantasy of intimacy. The woman who perceives conflict and feelings such as anger or resistance to closeness as an indication that a man is not loving is thwarting the possibility of a genuinely intimate relationship based on working through the real differences that exist.

Relating to him realistically means seeing beyond romantic notions of harmonious and conflict-free love and intimacy that cannot exist because of the inherent conditioned differences in men and women.

Other Realities

After the Romantic Beginning, What to Expect: Actions and Reactions

As one partner moves in one defensive direction, the other moves in the opposite direction.

1. Women who overly romanticize their relationships ("love too much") will experience their partner pulling away, becoming emotionally distant, and focused externally. She feels as though he is withdrawing his love and rejecting her, but this is only an unconscious reaction to the imbalance in involvement.
2. Women who emotionalize in extreme ways will eventually feel that their partner is angry, cold, distant, and uncaring. As she gets "hotter," his response gets "colder."
3. Women who have self-esteem problems (feelings of being unworthy) will experience their partner as discounting them, being abusive, and acting selfishly.
4. Women who have difficulty maintaining their separate identity and boundaries will experience their partners as controlling. A vacuum is created that he fills unconsciously.
5. Women who become fearful, and unable to cope when conflict or arguments arise will experience their partner as impatient, threatening, and frightening. This is due in part to a defensively fearful reaction on the

woman's part, causing her to see the man as being dangerous or "out of control."

6. Women who have trouble making decisions and expressing themselves will experience their partner as taking them for granted and being insensitive to their wishes. A man's compulsion to act and take responsibility is intensified by a woman's resistance to it.
7. Women who need reassurance of love due to their own insecurity will experience their partner as cold, selfish, and rejecting as a defense against the pressure to give what he can't.
8. Women who have a continuing need to analyze and discuss the relationship will experience their partner as closed off and basically incommunicative. Men become silent to counter a demand for communication they can't fulfill.
9. Women who become totally immersed in the home and children to the exclusion of involvement in the outside world will experience their partner as "a workaholic or busy," tired, emotionally withdrawn, and disinterested in the relationship. To the degree that women cut themselves off from the outside world, men become obsessed by it.

The principle in all of the preceding items is that women who move to one extreme in the relationship are part of the process that unconsciously polarizes their partner into the opposite extreme. Women are equal players in the cycles generated and have equal power to lessen or increase the polarization. It is impossible to separate out who is the real cause of the polarization cycle. The cycle is to blame for the pain and miscommunication.

Without a mutual change process or rebalancing, engaged in reciprocally by both partners, one's partner may begin to seem like a psychotic monster in a growing nightmare. Eventually, almost any new and reasonably attractive person will seem desirable and be experienced as a refuge from the pain and frustration of the relationship.

Conversely, the relationship will be ready for improvement and healing when there is the recognition and acknowledgment of being in a mutually polarizing process that can be transformed by the efforts of each partner who focuses on his or her equal responsibility in its creation.

Relating to him realistically means that expecting or pressuring for change on his side of this polarization cycle without an equal focus on her role in this process is guaranteed not only to exacerbate the problem but to create a growing negative perception of the partner as being unloving and destructive.

Critical Realities: Recognizing When His Relationship Behavior Is Nothing Personal

1. *In an honest relationship, conflict will appear early on and will be intense—but will diminish with time as greater intimacy evolves with each resolved conflict.*

In a traditionally romantic relationship, there will be very little if any conflict in the beginning, and things will seem magically mutual and loving. Suddenly, however, things will seem to deteriorate as denied conflict and anger emerge just when a real relationship is beginning.

2. *If he's a real person and not a man hiding behind smooth pretenses, he will have difficulty with, and anxiety about, intimacy and openness at the beginning of the relationship. However, once he feels it is safe to give himself over to it and that he is not being manipulated or used as an object to satisfy a woman's needs, he will be able to develop a strong attachment and intense involvement.*

If he is a "magical man," arriving on the energy of a romantic fantasy, wonderful intimacy will seem to exist from the start. The best will come first, however. The magical "closeness" will dissipate and prove shallow and brittle, until the relationship finally evaporates.

Easily achieved, intense intimacy with a man is defensive, false, and filled with denial of reality. Real intimacy is achieved slowly and through an acknowledgment that conflict is inevitable and must be mutually worked through.

3. *When a relationship first hits troubled waters and becomes polarized, traditional men will resist change, introspection, and communication.*

He feels hopeless about making his feelings known without either making matters worse or finding himself blamed. Therefore, "There's really nothing to talk about," will be his response.

The woman who does not press for openness, intimacy, and reassurance while a man is struggling to understand the situation, will facilitate his tentative movement toward intimacy and "opening up."

Men who don't open up, sense a danger in doing so. Therefore, pressing for "openness" will prove counterproductive, serving to increase his sense of danger and causing him to withdraw even more. Men "open up" when they feel it's truly safe to do so.

4. *Once a man is committed to a relationship, women have great potential power in it.*

The elements of a woman's power include men's tendency to feel guilty and inadequate about their personal relating skills. Also, a man's isolation creates dependency for happiness and fulfillment on the woman with whom he is involved. She becomes the sole focus for his personal needs, and losing her subjects him to his personal isolation and disconnection once more.

With an awareness and sensitivity to a man's experience in a relationship, developing a long-lasting, stable relationship with him is *not* difficult. Once involved, men need and want to remain in the relationship of their choice. Only the tension, frustration, and grinding-down effect of the *avoidable* polarization process causes a man to detach from his partner. With an awareness of her part in the cycle, a loving relationship can readily be sustained or restored.

5. *A man's negative, cynical, or self-protective attitudes exist in direct relationship to his externalization.*

The man's negative responses to life are a projection of his defensiveness. Confronting him with that and pressuring him to experience the world in a more positive way alienates him, because it fails to take into account the deeply rooted causes of his negative views of reality.

As a relationship balances, and the woman's dependence on him lessens, a man's "negative" perceptions may change because he feels less responsible for her and not as alone in his struggles. As a result, he may become less self-protective and preoccupied with external security in the form of work and finances, and more energy can be focused on the relationship.

6. *Making a relationship with a man the primary foundation of a woman's fulfillment and security plays into men's sense of feeling solely "responsible" for her happiness. This has two destructive side effects. It causes him to see himself as unrealistically powerful and potentially destructive if he is unsuccessful, and to hide those things about himself that he thinks might upset and make her unhappy. This will*

increase the likelihood of his withdrawing and becoming silent.

7. *Men's fear and anger toward women are comparable to women's fear and anger toward men, only in men it is expressed through withdrawal and resistance to intimacy and interaction. Men close up when they feel negative emotions, whereas women tend to open up and push for involvement.*

8. *To negotiate conflict with a man, give him specifics and in discussion stay close to the issue. Otherwise, most men give up in exasperation because their need for logic and objectivity is frustrated. Conflict will escalate.*

9. *Expect the following from men in the process of committing and becoming close:*

    a. Love expressed by being protective, taking responsibility, and "doing" for his partner.
    b. Confusion in him between love and feeling responsibility, so that he feels love as he also is made to feel responsible and guilt-ridden.
    c. Intense attachment and dependency (possessiveness) once he has committed himself to the relationship.
    d. Resistance to listening because his sense of feeling responsible puts him in pursuit of "answers" during any dialogue. In conversation he is thinking about solving the problems dis-

cussed, and providing answers for the questions.

10. *You are who you attract. Relating to a man realistically means recognizing that your initial attraction to him was not a mistake or an accident, but a reflection of who and what you are also. A healthy starting point in gaining understanding and improvement in a relationship involves identifying your inner needs that caused you to be attracted to him.*

Interaction Realities

Some Responses in Women that Trigger His Worst Relationship Tendencies

1. When a woman who won't make decisions or take action, then becomes angry over feeling controlled when the man does.
2. When a woman continues a discussion after a man pleads with her to stop talking.
3. When a woman accuses a man of being intentionally hurtful and uncaring once he has committed himself to the relationship and has broken off from other women.
4. When a woman pursues relationship talk when a man's focus is clearly elsewhere, and then accuses him of not caring because he doesn't respond or seems distracted.
5. When a woman asks a man for openness

and honesty, then responds with tears and anger when he exposes true feelings.
6. When a woman asks a man to spend more time with her and then provides no input about how that time will be spent.
7. When a woman is attracted to a man for the work he does and then resents his involvement with it and accuses him of using his work to neglect and avoid her.

Elusive Realities: "He's Not Doing That." Separating What You Feel He's Doing from What He Believes He's Doing

One man reported the following: "We are talking about investments, about which I have twenty-five years' experience and Irene has almost none. When I offered her what I felt was good and well-intentioned advice, I noticed her becoming angry at me and I asked her what was wrong. She said I sounded patronizing and was talking to her like a child. I explained, but she seemed unwilling to believe or accept the possibility that I did not have that feeling about her and that I was really happy to be sharing information I felt would help her. After that experience of miscommunication I could feel myself closing up and becoming cautious about everything I said to her because I could never be sure how she would interpret my motives."

Similarly, a businessman, after a lunch with his fiancée, became distracted because of a very important business meeting he had scheduled. He found himself accused of taking his future wife for granted and of being bored with her. "I knew right then that we had some serious problems, even though this seemed like a minor argument. It made me realize that in spite of her saying how much she loved me, she didn't really know me or trust my love. Who is she in love with, I thought to myself, if she thinks so badly of me?"

Relating to him realistically means separating out a woman's interpretation of a man's intentions from what he says he feels and intends. When a woman feels criticized, rejected, distanced, used, or patronized, she must at least consider the possibility that her partner has not intentionally set out to make her feel this way, and that by accusing him, she will only trigger a defensive reaction.

Men close off and withdraw when they find themselves accused and unable to make their motivations known and believed.

Early in relationships, many women tend to see nonexistent virtues in men. After romance, they perceive nonexistent unloving, negative intentions. Often the relationship ends without her ever having truly related to the "him" that he knows himself to be.

Therefore, relating to him realistically means separating out when:

a. He's not doing it at all but a woman believes he is due to her insecurities.

b. When he is doing it but it has become significantly magnified in impact because of a woman's insecurities.
c. He is doing it but it is unintentional.
d. He is doing it but he's responding in the way he automatically responds to everyone, in which case constructive, rather than defensive feedback about his actions is needed.

Do You Really Want a Successful Man?

It is self-defeating for a woman to be attracted to a man because of his ambition, only to feel rejected and resentful once a relationship with him has begun, because the focus of his energies continues in the direction they were in when they first met. The ambitious, driven man is unconsciously riveted to his goals and driven by his anxieties. His energies cannot be readily divided between his partner and his work, simply by an act of conscious intention. Many successful men try and fail in this endeavor.

Women attracted to externalized, goal-oriented men need to recognize that this unconscious process cannot easily be changed, and in fact is likely to intensify with time. Women who become committed to such men need to recognize the personal limitations and struggles inherent in such a relationship, because the components of his success drive include:

An external goal focus
A competitive orientation
An analytical or intellectual approach to problems
A controlling, ego-centered style
An autonomous, enclosed, self-protective posture of not needing anyone
A tendency to manipulate people and situations to gain advantage

The more driven the man, the greater the degree that the preceding traits exist and the more they will interfere with his capacity for emotional, intimate involvement in a personal relationship.

To presume that a man can simply alter his priorities is a tantalizing illusion and one that is unrealistic and destructive to the relationship. Many women believe that it is simply a matter of intention and desire on the man's part, and that if he "really wanted to," and if he "really cared," he could give more of himself to the relationship. This generates anger and hurt in women who feel they are treated insensitively by the self-absorbed, success-driven man.

Marriages between women and successful men are frequently experienced negatively, accompanied by intense feelings of anger and pain by the women. Inevitably he will be seen as self-centered, distant, controlling, insensitive, and manipulative. The man feels misunderstood and bewildered by such an interpretation of his motives, because he is convinced that he is acting in responsible, loving ways.

Loving Him as He Wants to Be Loved

Because the starting point for genuine intimacy with a man is the experience of the man himself, love and closeness are a fragile fantasy when they are based on only one person's needs and feelings, without knowing the inner reality of the other. If the reality of a man is offensive or negative, then a woman's love for him is as limited as the love that a man expresses toward a woman who feels unknown and used by him.

To love a man as he really is, or as he wants to be loved, may be too much to ask, but acknowledging the limitations and the struggle of both sexes to know and like each other as people, becomes more workable. It frees the relationship from the defeating, distorted interpretations that make it seem as though men alone bear the responsibility for being insensitive and unloving.

To love him as he is, or wants to be loved, is to avoid distorting or reacting critically to his loving intentions; to avoid lumping him into stereotyped and sexist categories; to avoid expecting responses from him that he *cannot* give because of his conditioning; and to avoid placing unfair blame on him for things that go wrong in the relationship.

I have spoken to hundreds of men about their ideas of intimacy and connection with women. I distilled from their input the key elements they articulated. I conclude this book with some composite quotes about what men want and need.

- "A woman who is able to hear and accept what I tell her is her impact on me without her reacting defensively and telling me that I am critical or unloving. I'd like her instead to use what I tell her to bring us closer together."
- "A woman who is in touch with and can acknowledge openly her 'darker egocentric motives' so that I'm not the only one described as the one being self-centered and exploiting the opposite sex.

  "I want her to see and recognize the limitations of her loving; the way that she uses me and loves me in a self-serving way and for her to acknowledge the deeper negative feelings and images she has about men and relationships."
- "When we argue or experience conflict and tension, and talk about it, I want a woman who wants first to know how she contributed to triggering my negative or 'bad reactions' so that I know that she is sensitive to the two-way street of our communication. I don't want to be told that I'm the one with problems and hostility, and that I can't love."
- "A woman whose love for me is based on the me I know myself to be, and not the 'wonderful me' of her imagination. I don't want to have to live up to her romantic fantasies of me and her image of me as being different from other men. I am bound to fail at living up to that, and I'm sure to disappoint her."
- "A woman who can feel good about me and

the relationship without inflating it, or making it a lopsided emphasis, to the exclusion of all the other things in her life—socially and otherwise. If she inflates the relationship, I feel pressured to give it more than I want to, and when I can't, I feel like I'm the spoiler. In other words, I want a woman who can see and accept the limits of our interaction as well as our potential, without feeling that less intensity on my part is bad or diminishes the good we have."

- "I want a woman who will allow me my view of the world without telling me I have to change because I'm warped and negative."
- "A woman who will fight it out with me and when we argue can see our differences as a part of our struggle to get closer, not as something bad that means I have damaged the relationship because I've expressed my conflicts about it."
- "A woman who will not make me responsible for her happiness beyond what I am and can do in the relationship. Nor do I want her to sacrifice any of what she is for me and make me responsible for filling the vacuum it creates."
- "A woman who not only can tell me what she doesn't like about us, but can provide specific alternatives that we can work on together. I don't want to be responsible for reading her mind or coming up with solutions that make her happy. It's not enough to be told about what I do that doesn't work or feel good. I want to know what does work and what will feel good to her that I'm capable of doing."

- "I want a woman who values the work I do, even if it seems as if I do it to satisfy my own ego. I don't want what I do to be interpreted negatively, and what I don't seem to do well to be made crucial and the cause of our problems."
- "A woman who will give to me what I value and desire, not what she decides is loving and valuable, and that I should want."
- "A woman who doesn't see me either as a superman or a jerk but as a flawed, struggling, limited person; capable in some areas and incompetent in others and as vulnerable in my way as she is in hers."

I believe that as women understand and come to grips with the unique struggle and experience of men, and the way that both sexes have been impaired by traditional conditioning and interactions, that a doorway through which both sexes can move toward a new, mutually fulfilling reality can be opened. This unpolarized pathway can liberate and facilitate the healthiest and most constructive life experience for both sexes. That is my understanding of the psychology of the sexes, my vision of our mutual potential, and my hope for a psychological evolution that will ultimately free us from some of the dark and destructive psychological forces that have traditionally transformed exciting beginnings into destructive endings.